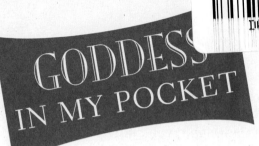

GODDESS
IN MY POCKET

GODDESS
IN MY POCKET

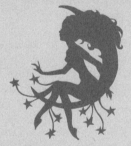

Simple Spells, Charms, Potions, and Chants
TO GET YOU EVERYTHING YOU WANT

Patricia Telesco

HarperSanFrancisco
A Division of HarperCollins*Publishers*

HarperCollins Web Site: http: //www.harpercollins.com

HarperCollins®, ▉®, and HarperSanFrancisco™ are trademarks of HarperCollins Publishers Inc.

HarperCollins books may be purchased for educational, business, or sales promotional use. For information please write: Special Markets Department, HarperCollins Publishers, Inc., 10 East 53rd Street, New York, NY 10022.

FIRST EDITION

Library of Congress Cataloging-in-Publication Data
Telesco, Patricia.
        Goddess in my pocket : simple spells, charms, potions, and chants to get you everything you want / Patricia Telesco. — 1ˢᵗ ed.
ISBN 0–06–251550–0 (pbk.)
1. Charms. 2. Incantations. 3. Magic. 4. Aphrodisiacs. 5. Goddess religion. I. Title.
        BF 1621.T43   1998
        133.4'4—dc21   97–52608

98 99 00 01 02 RRDH 10 9 8 7 6 5 4 3 2 1

To the Goddess.

From your dewdrops and starlight

I have found the essence of true magic growing in my heart

Also: for

Jeremy, Samantha, and Karl with love.

★

MAGIC IN THE OFFICE   57

★

MAGIC ON THE ROAD   83

★

MAGIC IN RELATIONSHIPS   117

★

MAGIC IN YOUR POCKET   152

INTRODUCTION

*A little in one's own pocket is better
than much in another man's purse.*
— MIGUEL DE CERVANTES

Ever feel like you could use a little magic in your life? To spice up
your sex life or tone down daily stress? To juggle the chaos or balance your checkbook? To attract lovers or repel thorny problems?
Consider this: we all have a world full of modern magic at our disposal, the Goddess in our pockets, so to speak. We just have to
learn how to reach inside ourselves and draw out her sacred energy.

The key to doing this is to stop thinking about spirituality as
something reserved for funerals, weddings, or door-to-door mission-
aries. Our spiritual nature, that internal goddess, is always with us.
When we let her, this goddess can become a powerful partner for
taking action in our lives. The purpose of this book is to give you the
tools necessary to begin reclaiming that partnership with the
Goddess's magic in one hand and a good sense of humor in the other.

Looking to the Goddess for insights and personal empower-
ment is nothing new. It's been going on ever since humankind first

turned to faith as a way of resolving life's problems and mysteries. From ensuring abundant harvests to curing the sniffles to establishing a relationship between star-crossed lovers, our ancestors used every means at their disposal—material or mystical—to improve their quality of life.

While times have changed, our need for the Goddess's help certainly has not. Thankfully, her tradition of magic remains with us, reminding us that a divine thread shapes our life and holds it together even when circumstances try to yank the fibers apart. Better still, this thread is not intangible and unknowable; it is within each human being just waiting to be rediscovered.

Have no doubts! Each of us is part Goddess. Yes, you too, fellas! When you look in the mirror first thing in the morning it might seem difficult, if not downright absurd, to think of yourself as divine or mystical in any way. Getting stuck in traffic, changing diapers, managing budgets, racing to get dinner on the table—none of this makes us feel particularly divine or enlightened. Yet, even flossing our teeth can be magical if we allow it to be (consider the potential symbolism in a spell focused on loosening up a sticky situation!). This may seem far-fetched at first, but familiarity is exactly what will energize your magic! Being able to immediately recognize symbolism helps in willfully directing magical energy. And don't underestimate the power of humor. Joy is one of the most incredible magics on earth.

Most people could use a little guidance in finding the Goddess in themselves and activating her energy effectively in everyday activities. That's exactly where this book can help. Whether you want to regain control of your life by using metaphysical reigns or just sprinkle a little extra magical glitter on your day, pick up this guide. In it you'll find dozens of amulets, charms, and other potent portables to make life a little happier, a little easier, and a lot more fun.

Bright blessings!

GODDESS

IN MY POCKET

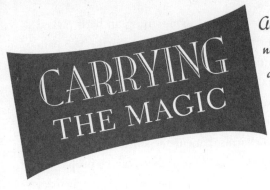

CARRYING THE MAGIC

Aim at the sun. You may not reach it, but your arrow will fly far higher than if aimed at an object on a level with yourself.

—J. HAWES

"Who, me?" This is the most common response I get from people when I tell them that true magic, and the spark of the Goddess, already lies within each of us. We carry it all the time. It is part of what makes each person wonderfully quirky and unique. This means that the most important factor in working effective magic anywhere, anytime, is not a "hip" robe or funky crystal jewelry, but *you*. Okay, take a deep breath and let this revelation sink in. Once you get over the shock and realize that true magic lies within yourself, learning how to facilitate magical power will be much easier.

Finding ways to enable magic in any setting is a tradition as old as dirt, a tradition that was started by people who didn't have the local quickie-mart to rely on for daily necessities. So, when someone had a headache, instead of buying aspirin, he or she would invoke the Goddess's power through a spell, an empowered potion, or an herb picked during a waning moon—using an herb picked when the moon was "shrinking" was thought to make the pain shrink. Few of us have time for hour-long rituals or eloquent invocations, but this simple magic, which has worked effectively for centuries, could serve us all well.

The wizardry of the ancients frequently included the making of amulets, talismans, and charms that enhanced the bearer's power in the world or provided protection. One of these, which people still use, is the lucky rabbit's foot. Other examples of ancient wizardry include wearing certain colors and scents, or repeating superstitious actions to control the seemingly senseless whims of fate. And if you think we've grown beyond such things, just look at the modern practices of color and aroma therapy, or at those of us who knock on wood and cross our fingers for luck, just in case!

Since the Goddess's magic is not about to disappear anytime soon (she's a very persistent lady), this book acts a guide to making a modern metaphysical medicine kit: fashioning spells, choosing accoutrements, and enacting mini-rituals to release metaphysical energy into our lives, no matter where we may be. In this chapter you will become familiar with these tools and techniques, so you can tailor-make any magical procedure to effectively meet your needs and goals. As you read, remember that the implied magic here begins in your mind and heart—with the belief that *you* really do have the power to change your life.

I Think I Can, I Think I Can!

Before you contemplate any magical procedures, you need to get rid of tendencies toward self-doubt, which also leads to self-defeat. The phrases "I can't" or "I'm not sure" really don't fit into the Goddess's lingo. It is one thing to recognize our limits and another altogether to *create* limits based on residual teenage angst or adult insecurities. Too many of us underestimate the power of the human mind and spirit to manifest tangible changes.

To make magic a reality, instead of just wishful thinking, we have to accept that there is much more to life, and to our own minds, than the supposed concrete "truths." Magic is part of the immaterial, which we can see manifested in those miraculous moments and bits of insight that defy pat, cookie-cutter explanations. It is long past time to believe in ourselves as powerful co-creators—with the Goddess—of our destiny. We also need to begin acting on that conviction.

Remember the "little engine that could"? If you believe you can, *you can!* Embrace a little bit of childlike faith and you'll find the Goddess's magic in the treasure chest of your heart, just waiting for you to unlock it.

A Pocket Full of Miracles

Just because magic begins with childlike faith doesn't mean that logical, adult insights have no place in metaphysics. Conscious, rational thought processes help with magical planning, first by evaluating the basic situation. What's going on? What exactly do I want? What type of magical procedure is most suited to achieving my goal without arousing the neighbors' overactive imagination? What symbolic components can I use to complete the procedure?

It's hard to answer these questions without first knowing exactly what each process entails. That's where this section will help. The following are descriptions, in alphabetical order, of the objects and techniques used in this book. Become familiar with these, so that when you go to pull the Goddess's energy out of your pocket, you'll know exactly what procedure to grab and how to use it effectively.

AMULET:

An amulet is a preservative—that is, something worn as a remedy or protection against evil. Common ancient amulets included stones, metals, hides, or plants with special words, phrases, or images inscribed on them. The St. Christopher medal is a good modern example that travelers still use for protection. Another example is the two-part Mitzpah coin. Two lovers each carry one-half of the coin to protect them while they're apart and ensure their devotion.

According to early experts, amulets worked best when made during a propitious moon sign, hour, weekday, and so forth. This can get rather burdensome for modern work-a-day folk. So, I suggest creating amulets whenever you wish, and I recommend adding symbolic timing when your schedule will allow. While timing does add another dimension to your magical methodology, and I recommend optimal timing periodically throughout this book, don't feel bound by it. Much more important than *when* you make an amulet is *that* you make it.

CHARGING:

Charging is a way of activating any object's latent magical potential for a specific goal—and you need not have a Visa or MasterCard to do it! This process is very similar to giving a battery a jump start. You place an object in moonlight, sunlight, water, or rich soil to gather the energy of that medium. Moonlight is a good choice for magic centering on the intuitive nature, while sunlight has a conscious, active principle. Water is soothing, refreshing, and healing; earth, grounded and growth-oriented. While there are other ways of magically empowering objects, these four work fairly universally for any charm, amulet, talisman, or fetish you might design.

CHARM:

A charm can be one of two things. First, it can be an empowered word or symbol that evokes a magical response, often in matters of love. Frequently this form of charm is uttered, like an incantation, taking its meaning from the Latin *carmen,* meaning song or poem.

Giving traditional charms a face-lift is not difficult. Most people already understand the power of words. We just have to learn to give specific magical potency to our speech. Consider the effect angry words have on a listener. That's because there's real *energy* propelling them. In working on verbal charms, think of that kind of power, but without the negativity.

A charm can also be very similar to an amulet. This object is worn on a person in the hope of improving fortune and averting evil. Ever wonder what all those trinkets in a charm bracelet were for? Well, now you know! Some examples are a tiny heart for love, an anchor for security or safety at sea, baby shoes for fertility, and a clover for luck.

To my mind, the best way to make a charm is to combine the two definitions: begin with an object symbolic of your desire, then fortify that object with magical energy, using words and phrases, such as chants and incantations.

FETISH:

Unlike the obsessions or fixations we usually think of as fetishes, magical fetishes have nothing to do with kinky sex, unless contrived for that purpose. In magic, fetishes are closely related to charms, getting their name from the Latin word *facere*, "to make." A fetish can be any natural or created object that arouses a strong emotional response, specifically a feeling that the object represents or holds a higher power.

For example, when you get pulled over by the police and they flash a badge, the natural reaction is to wonder what we have done wrong. The badge represents an authority or power that evokes an immediate emotional response. In a magical setting this might be a carving of the Goddess, or some other meaningful object, that is used in rituals or as a focus in spell casting to invoke divine energy.

INCANTATION:

Taking its meaning from the Latin word *incantare*, which means "to chant a magical formula," an incantation is a verbal or mental magical formula that specifies your desire to the Goddess. Incantations focus the energy of a spell or ritual, and they sometimes invoke spirits or the Goddess for aid.

Verbalized incantations carry the energy of our intentions through tones and vibrations. When propriety won't allow for this, there is nothing wrong with mentally reciting the words of a spell. Let's face it—most of us can't just start chanting at the office or around our grandmothers!

In historical texts, many incantations rhyme. Rhyming helped the illiterate people of that time to memorize a spell (through oral tradition), but it is not necessary for a spell to work. So when you create your own incantations, don't worry if you can't come up with Shakespearean-styled verses, or ones that rhyme! What's most important about an incantation is that it helps you concentrate on the magic, that it's specific, and that it guides the energy toward its goal.

INTERNALIZATION:

Internalizing the energy of a spell means to accept it as part of your everyday life and actions. When you work magic for love, start expecting it and begin loving yourself; when you work magic for joy, do things that can encourage that lighthearted spirit, like watching funny movies.

My personal favorite way to internalize any magic is by creating edible components. This way you truly "are what you eat"! Then again, as a militant "kitchen witch," I advocate any good excuse to make tantalizing magical meals. It's fun, flavorful, and filling!

INVOCATION:

To invoke means to call for assistance, specifically the assistance of the Goddess through prayer. Don't let the idea of praying put you off. It's nothing more than a heartfelt request that you put before the divine. So, stop thinking about the King James Bible or phrases with the word *forsooth,* and just *talk* to the Goddess. She cares far less about *what* you say than *why* you say it. Use slang, rap, or whatever form of communication works best for you.

MEDITATION, VISUALIZATION:

Meditation and visualization usually work together in magical settings. Meditation is a way of thinking deeply about something, and mulling it over completely in your mind from as many different angles as possible. Visualization adds a second dimension to this process. In visualization a person imagines all the circumstances of a particular subject, making a mental movie out of it. From this perspective, many people find they gain emotional distance and, therefore, a much better understanding of what's going on.

For the purpose of this book, meditation and visualization direct the energy of a spell more specifically. Think of this as readying a spiritual bow and taking aim with thoughts. Magic works through willpower; meditation in combination with visualization hones that will, focuses it intently, then helps release the power to hit your mark.

SPELL:

In Anglo-Saxon the word for spell is *spelung,* meaning to turn or change. Magically speaking, you will be using spells to turn or change the life-energy that exists all around us and then activate it to achieve a specific goal. Most spells include some type of written or verbal charm (or prayer) that empowers and directs the magic. When writing or chanting aren't possible, simply concentrate in detail on the spell's purpose.

Unlike in *Macbeth,* you won't find any tongue of frog or eye of newt as spell components in this book. "Pocket magic" uses ingredients that are fairly available around your living space, the supermarket, or dollar store, or those that fill the shelves at New Age outlets. Why? Because using unfamiliar ingredients in spell casting hinders the flow of magic. The more meaning each component has for you, the better it works!

TALISMAN:

Like charms and amulets, a talisman preserves the bearer from misfortune. A talisman is a figure created under auspicious astrological conditions to energize it for a specific purpose. Frequently this figure is carved on sympathetic metals and stones to amplify its power. Since this could prove very difficult unless you know an engraver or lapidary, many talismans suggested in this book consist of symbols written or painted on paper or cloth.

Throughout the book I provide examples of talismans for achieving numerous needs and goals, as well as procedures for creating them. Even so, I highly encourage you to use your personal vision and creativity as a guide in fashioning your own portable magics. In the process, I think you'll find that you intuitively know a lot more about the Goddess's magic than you might have thought. So, turn your pockets inside out and see what wonders they hold!

Putting It All Together

Once you've decided which object or technique is best suited to your magical goal, you can begin the process of choosing and gathering your ingredients. Imagine you are making a mystical salad. You're going to mix 'n' match various elements for a fulfilling and potent blend, using the Goddess's magic as "dressing."

The potential elements you can use for pocket magic are nearly limitless. But when you feel lost for ideas, check out the suggestions given under the Alternative Components sections in this book. These, combined with the sample spells and the information that follows, should inspire your imagination when you choose components for personalized magic.

AROMATICS, HERBS, FLOWERS, AND TREES:

There is very little, if anything, on this planet that hasn't been used at least once for magical purposes. Our ancestors believed that nature acted as the Goddess's mirror—that they could discover her reflection and power in the world, and in themselves, if they looked closely enough. I agree wholeheartedly.

Nature provides us with the most diversified tools that anyone could hope for. In pocket magic, aromatics improve our mental state and focus by subtly nudging our awareness with their scents. Plant parts can become spell components, amulets, charms, fetishes, wands to direct your energy, or even divination media. In other words, anything natural goes with magic like bread goes with butter. Just make sure that the item's symbolic value corresponds with your intentions. You don't want to use a plant associated with banishing when casting love spells!

The symbolism you associate with an aromatic, flower, spice, or tree can come from either the traditional correspondences provided in magical texts or your personal experience. I believe the latter is preferable, but some folks are just more secure in trusting "expert" opinions. Again, approach this however you feel most comfortable.

COLOR MAGIC:

Psychology has shown that color affects humans tremendously. In pocket magic, colors symbolize intentions. Metaphysically and mentally, colors act as a cue to our subconscious, will, and superconscious (the spiritual nature that connects us with, and communicates with, the greater powers), reinforcing and focusing energy more specifically.

Using symbolic colors for pocket magic isn't necessary, but it is helpful and marvelously discreet. For example, while you might not be able to wear a fetish bag designed to ease stress openly at the office, you *can* don a specially blessed blue shirt, representing peace and tranquillity. In this case, clothes really do make the person!

To choose a color, consider how it makes you feel and what words come immediately to mind when you see it. Red usually represents energy, strength, and vitality; blue, restfulness and the clearing of troubles; orange, the harvest and friendship; yellow, creativity and mental functions; white, protection and purity; green, growth and healing; and purple, spirituality and leadership.

CRYSTALS, ROCKS, AND MINERALS:

You can hardly walk into a department store these days without seeing crystal pendants, geode bookends, and the like. The fascination with stones of all kinds has certainly not been limited to this decade—just look at the pet rocks of the 1970s, or the Language of Stones of the 1870s! No matter the time period, humans have always loved their baubles. In magic, rather than use them just decoratively, we also put these bits of earth to work.

Crystals have a natural ability to hold energy (quartz being a prime example). So, they can be used in spells, charms, amulets, talismans, and fetishes, with as many diverse applications as other natural objects. There are many different stones, shells, metals, and minerals, each with its magical correspondences, but the color and shape of each provides some potential symbolism right away. A red stone that is roughly shaped like a heart would make an excellent charm for improved relationships, for example, whereas a blue-tinted seashell could be energized to help you "circumnavigate," or "go with the flow," through a difficult situation.

FOODS AND BEVERAGES:

Foods and beverages can be used on altars as offerings to the Goddess. Since the ingredients for both often have magical associations, it's not surprising to find pocket magicians concocting a love potion, tossing a money salad, or baking providence bread. The only difference between this and making family dinners is the way you prepare the food or beverage, and what significance it has for you while it's being consumed.

Besides internalizing specific types of magical energy through digestion, enchanted foods and beverages can become portable magic in several ways. Dry, preserve, can, freeze, or bottle some and enjoy the magic later, when it's needed. Or, pack the magic for an empowering picnic or lunch.

SYMBOLS:

Magically speaking, a symbol is no less powerful than what it represents. Since you will be wearing or carrying some of these visibly, you will want your chosen magical symbols to be both as personally meaningful and as publicly palatable as possible.

If a symbol makes you think immediately about your goal or need, it's a good choice, be it a traditionally magical symbol or not. For example, we often think of a red cross as having to do with people's well-being, because of the organization it represents. So, a red cross could become part of a cross-stitch talisman for health, in which every knot binds the energy to the token. Or, more simply, if a woman wasn't feeling very well she might inscribe a cross on the afflicted area with red nail polish or lipstick, then wash it off to symbolically carry away the malady.

TIMING

Just as people venerate nature for depicting the Goddess's power, they also look to the heavens as representing her qualities. Different astrological signs, each phase of the moon, each day of the week, and every hour in the day can affect a magical procedure for boon or bane, depending on the attributes they emphasize. For example, a waning moon is considered a good time to create magical items for banishing negativity, so that the bad energy will shrink like the moon. Conversely, a spell cast by a waxing moon or full moon brings positive growth and maturity.

With everyone being so busy these days, it's very difficult to follow precise timing guidelines. If you have some leeway in your schedule, and the need is not overly pressing, I suggest consulting a good astrological calendar for help in timing your magic. Otherwise, let your inner voice and urgency guide you.

MISCELLANEOUS ITEMS:

Miscellaneous items include all the wonders of technology and the interesting additions to our lives that the ancients never imagined possible. Take paper clips as an example. We don't read about the ancient Egyptians using "papyrus clips" as magical symbols. But if paper clips *had* been invented then, you can bet a creative pocket magician would have used them to symbolize connections and staying power!

This is one area where your magic can get really creative. Use staples in a medicine bag to help hold a relationship together, or two pieces of a heart bound with glue stick to engender devotion. The possibilities are as limitless as your imagination!

THE GODDESS:

As the magical matron of this book, the Goddess is essential to everything we hope to achieve. In each section of this book I give the names of goddesses from around the world and explore the attributes of each in a magical setting. Why? Because the Goddess represents the creative vital force of the universe—part of which energizes and guides magic.

As "prodigal children" of this creative force, the more we connect with the Goddess externally, the easier it becomes to see that we carry her power within, too. It is but one short step from this astonishing realization to seeing our lives transform in ways that seem miraculous. The amazement we feel at this doesn't constitute a lack of faith in the Goddess's magic or our personal abilities. It's natural to feel awestruck when everything "works"—in awe of the Sacred Parent, in awe of her spark within us—and in awe of the magic created when the human factor and the divine combine harmoniously.

Alongside these elements, don't forget to use healthy doses of practicality and personal vision. If you have a different image of the Goddess you want to call upon, other components you want to use, or another way of achieving the same magical ends that's more meaningful to you, do so! As the old saying goes, "If it ain't broke, don't fix it." Just do what works for you.

The Pocket Magician's Kit

In the beginning of this chapter I talked
about making a magic kit of sorts.
Since we live in a very mobile society, it's nice to have a small,
portable kit filled with flexible
components that you enjoy. So,
stop at a secondhand shop
and find a small suitcase,
makeup box, toolbox, or
other container that has compartments or that you can
easily add compartments to.
Fill this with odds and ends
that you favor for magic, and
keep it in your car, purse, briefcase, suitcase, or wherever. This
way, when circumstances don't offer
suitable ingredients for your magic, you
can still pull what you need out of your
pocket (or pocketbook) with little fuss.

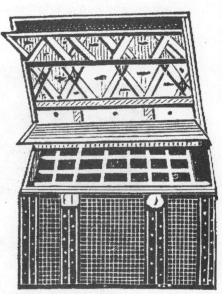

Help and Hints

After having practiced magic for well over a decade, I have gathered some insights and guidelines that will make your magical efforts more successful and fulfilling. First are the don'ts:

Don't try to work magic if you feel lousy, angry, or tired.

Don't try to manipulate anyone's free will. No matter how tempting it might seem, the results won't last and won't make you happy.

Don't work magic for anything that you're not willing to foster daily in word and deed (in other words, if you're going to "talk the talk," also "walk the walk").

And, finally, don't expect that magic will manifest exactly as you anticipate. The Universe has a wicked sense of humor and a completely different outlook than we do on what's best for us; trust me on this one.

ON THE OTHER HAND,

Do enact everything you can on a mundane level to support your magical goals.

Do individualize your magic, and begin by using personal items as components.

Do repeat magical procedures any time you feel the desire to empower your life, and reinforce any magic "in the works."

Last, but not least, *do* believe in yourself and in your ability to tap into the Goddess within.

ZAP! THERE'S THE MAGIC!

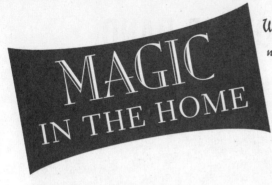

MAGIC IN THE HOME

Without hearts, there is no home.
—LORD BYRON

Hovel, hotel, or houseboat—your home should be your castle. If it's not, a little magic fairy dusting is in order. Of all the places where the Goddess can manifest herself, your home is one where she can really shine without the aid of furniture polish. Every part of your living space has magical potential. What about your living room, you ask? Use the TV screen as a crystal ball (but turn it off first)! And the rugs—metaphysically sweep problems under them!

One of the favorite magical jokes in my home is about the hot tub. When people come over and meet Trish the witch for the first time, we often open the tub by way of hospitality. A little later, when everyone's relaxed, I come out with a handful of mixed vegetables, a wooden spoon, and a sneaky grin! Gives a whole new meaning to "bubble, bubble," eh? The point is that the hot tub *could* be my cauldron if I wanted it to be, just as many things around your home can take on the Goddess's glimmer if you will allow them to.

Pantry Protection

Any home feels more comfy, cozy, and "cosmic" when it has magical protection to keep negativity in check. When safeguarding your home, it's a good idea to use things that already reside in that space. This way, friends and family who don't find magic "user friendly" won't notice the adjustments.

The Greek goddess Hera makes a good pantry protectress. She's a born fighter, bearing a sickle in one hand that she uses to safeguard homes and families. She is also the goddess of stability and security, two things that the word *home* immediately brings to mind.

PEARLS OF WISDOM (ONIONS, THAT IS):

In folk remedies, onions are used to draw out infections. This fetish uses that symbolism to draw out other figurative problems. Take a handful of pearl onions (skins intact) and string them on cotton thread. Allow them to dry, turning them regularly so they don't mold. Each time you turn the onions, repeat an empowering incantation like *"When I speak, let magic begin. What I command, be held within."* When the onions are completely dried, put them in a small drawstring bag near your stove.

Use the fetish when someone has it in for you, or when your home is filled with tension. To activate the magic, take out one onion. Name it after the problem you're experiencing, and focus wholly on that situation. To dispel the negativity, either burn the onion in your fireplace or throw it away in the trash.

You can carry one of the onions with you when you leave the house, too, as a charm to absorb spite, ire, and dissension.

SPICE IT UP:

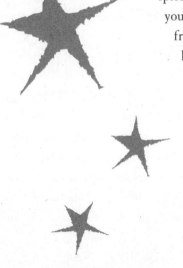

Want to give new meaning to the phrase "spice of life"? Look no farther than your kitchen spice rack. Take a cue from history: for centuries people have used common household spices for just about everything, including magic.

To safeguard your home, mix together a little powdered lemon rind (for cleansing), ginger (for energy), oregano (for love), and rosemary (for protection) with a cup of baking soda. This mixture can be used in several ways: sprinkle it counterclockwise around your living space to dispel or turn around negativity, then clean it up clockwise to attract positive energy; add the mixture to your wash water for regular magical maintenance; or put it in a pillow for your pet's bed to keep the creature healthy—an additional benefit here is that the mix acts as an effective deodorizer!

To turn this into portable power, just sprinkle the mixture in your shoes, and it will protect you wherever you go!

A SPELL "WORTH ITS SALT":

An old folk spell says that a pinch of salt placed under the chair of an unwelcome guest will get them to leave quickly. You might want to keep those door-to-door salespeople away by sprinkling salt over the threshold of your door.

For pocket magic, carry some salt with you to keep aggressive panhandlers and religious zealots at arm's length.

MAKE A CLEAN SWEEP:

Common household tools, brooms were also used by our ancestors for spiritual cleansing and protection. The modern magician might use a vacuum instead (hey, more power!): simply sweep or vacuum negativity and sickness *outward* from the center of your home, and then move inward to draw in positive energy.

For mobile magic? Carry a piece of broom to keep you safe.

QUARTER QUARTERS:

The cost of magically putting in your two cents' worth is about to increase. In magic, each of the four directions is called a Quarter. Many practitioners keep tokens at these points in their living space to safeguard the home and to attract the Goddess's energies to it. For this spell, you will need five quarters (those from the year of your birth are best). Hold them in your hands and visualize them being filled with brilliant, white light. Repeat the following phrase seven times (seven is the number of completion):

Earth and Air, Fire, and Sea,
come, ignite the magic in me.
North and South, East, and West,
by Hera's power, may this house always be blessed!

Continue the visualization until the coins feel hot in your hands. Put four of them in safe places, one each as close as possible to the four cardinal points in your living space. Retain the fifth as a portable protective charm to keep a little bit of home with you everywhere. And, hey, if need be you can always use it to "phone home."

Alternative Components:

For protection and to ensure pure intentions, use white napkins, tablecloths, or place mats. To keep out malintended magic, hang iron pans or copper-bottomed pans on the wall to "conduct" safety through the home. To wash away negativity, keep a pumice stone by your sink. All hot, spicy herbs, foods, and beverages like garlic, onions, clove, radishes, and rum will protect and purify your spirit from within. Trivets that feature brooms will sweep away problems.

If you are banishing troubles, work during a waning to dark moon, on Sundays, the sun's-day (so as to illuminate all shadows) during the month of January for defensive energy, or when the moon is in Aries for courage, or Pisces for endurance. Conversely, if you are trying to draw positive energy to your magic, work during the waxing to full moon, on Thursdays for increased power, during the month of March for overcoming problems, and when the moon is in Libra for harmony.

Kitchen Witches

Kitchen Witches are not just those little broom-flying dolls that you see in people's pantries. They are *real* people who enjoy making magic out of literally everything around their hearth. Nothing is safe from the creative kitchen witch's eye—from appliances and food to the dog's dish and pot holders! This section will give a whole new meaning to the idea of "stirring something up" in your kitchen.

Turning again to the Greeks for inspiration, the kitchen goddess is Hestia, the lady of the hearth, which is the heart of a living space. Hestia really keeps those home fires burning. She also represents duty, moderation, prudence, and patience, four things from which any home can benefit.

CUT THE CRAP:

Tired of some of the "b.s." around you? Wish that people would just get to the point instead of beating around the bush? This amulet is designed to help. Grab a grocery bag, and draw an image on it that somehow represents your present situation. Fold this image inward three times, then take a steak knife or kitchen scissors and begin cutting the image into nine pieces, saying as you cut,

Truth be told, words be bold,
as I work, the magic unfolds.

Gather the scraps together; set one aside and burn or bury the rest. Carry the remaining scrap with you, or put it up in a visible area to help manifest your will. When the magic comes to pass, burn this last scrap with a prayer of thanks.

CAN IT!

Need to get rid of a nagging problem, or make the best of a bad situation? Try canning it! Take a small empty can and put an image of your problem into it. Bury this in a pot of soil, and plant some flower seeds over it. By the time the plant sprouts, the difficulty should wane; when it flowers, all should be well. Then, dry and carry the flower petals as an amulet to keep that problem from returning.

An earth-friendly alternative to the can would be to make a biodegradable image of your difficulty, such as one carved out of a potato, and place it in the compost heap. Then nature can "do her thing" and slowly decompose the problem, turning the negative energy into something useful!

LIFE SUCKS LEMONADE:

You know the old saying "When life hands you lemons, make lemonade"? Energize this idea with magic! Begin by making lemonade from scratch. As you take each lemon, focus on the area of difficulty and literally put the squeeze on it. Retain the lemon peels. Stir the juice counterclockwise (to banish negativity), saying *"Gone, gone, gone, bad luck, be gone."* Focus your intention on turning things around, then begin stirring clockwise, saying *"Mine, mine, mine, all good things are mine."* Drink a sip of this three times a day, over three days; before sipping, repeat the last incantation three times. This supports the magic.

Keep a piece of the dried lemon rind with you as part of a medicine bag or fetish for protection. Grind up the rest to use in magical incense or cleansing solutions.

ABUNDANCE ON THE RISE:

When you need financial improvements, try baking bread. Begin with any frozen dough and add to it diced spinach, diced onion, a pinch of basil, and a little dill, all of which are associated with prosperity. While kneading in the vegetables and spices, concentrate on your need, saying,

> *Money to me, money to me,*
> *today I claim prosperity.*

Baking energizes the magic, and eating the bread internalizes the energy of abundance in your life. Even if money doesn't come right away, you won't have to buy a fresh loaf this week!

Gypsy lore says to place one piece of this bread in your pocket. This brings prosperity, luck, and providence.

Adjusting the herbs and incantation in this spell can make it into a spell to lift your spirits. To do this, add diced olives and a pinch of marjoram to the bread, and say something like

> *Sadness cease, joy released,*
> *cheer be free, inside of me.*

Carry a piece of this to maintain happiness.

CLEAN UP YOUR ACT:

To help rid yourself of a bad habit, wash it away with your dishes! Begin by drawing an emblem of the habit, using dish soap on as many of the plates, glasses, and other dishes as possible. Wash each dish counterclockwise to banish the tendency, while focusing wholly on your intention to change your life. Afterward, begin making positive efforts to achieve your goal. Repeat as often as needed, or until the dishes are done.

For pocket magic, carry one of the small sample bottles of dish soap as a gentle reminder of your goal. When you feel you need to reinforce the magic, use the soap to wash your hands, drawing the same emblem on them, then neatly rinsing it away.

STOP WINE-ING:

The great thing about kitchen magic is the fact that puns often help the energy along. Take a glass of wine in hand. Look into the glass and tell it all the sources of aggravation you currently have. You'll find it's a great listener. Stir the wine counterclockwise with the index finger of your strong hand, saying,

Away from me, all negativity.
When from this cup, wine pours, let joy be restored.

Pour out three-fourths of the wine on the ground, and let the soil neatly absorb the irritation. Turn your back and walk away. Do not look back.

Put the remaining wine in a small bottle, such as those from the airlines, and keep it with you. When other small nuisances arise, you can pour out the magic wherever you are!

THE STOVETOP CAULDRON:

This bit of magic brings continuity to any situation. Begin with a soup pot. Set out the ingredients for your favorite soup. Name the individuals or circumstances involved in the situation at hand as you cut up and place the ingredients in the pot. The heat creates the sympathetic congruity between these different aspects or people, and stirring clockwise draws positive energy to the situation. At this point, pray for Hestia's blessing. Pour off small helpings of the soup into sealed jars, and give one to each person involved in the situation. As they eat, they will internalize the power of harmony.

IT'S MY PANTRY AND I'LL SCRY IF I WANT TO:

Scrying is a form of divination that allows you to see symbolic or literal images in a specific medium as answers to questions. In the old days, scryers used a crystal, pond, or the sky. Today, your kitchen offers two easy alternatives: dish soap and creamer. If using dish soap, fill the sink with water, then add pearly soap to the top in a clockwise circle, thinking about a specific question as you pour. If using creamer, make your tea or coffee as usual, then pour in the creamer, also clockwise. Look at the shapes and images that form to discern the answer to your question. For example, if your query had to do with business, and a circle forms, this could mean that to attain your goal you'll need unity or a specific circle of people.

Alternative Components:

A lot here depends on your intent. For love, use red or pink knickknacks; for peacefulness, use amethyst, moonstone, or turquoise decorations. To attract specific energies, put magnets on the refrigerator (with an appropriate symbol, like an eye for insight, underneath them). For a little luck, try simmering cinnamon potpourri. Eat green foods for prosperity, and drink fruit juice for healthy energy.

Work during a full moon for manifestation, on Saturday to generate outcomes, during the month of May for progress, or when the moon is in Cancer for sensitivity.

Technological Wizardry

Magic seems almost anachronistic when we look at the wonders of space travel. Yet, what people once thought was magic has become today's reality. This means that technology and metaphysics can work together agreeably, especially for us "cool" spell casters who wouldn't be caught dead without our modern toys.

For technological wizardry, turn to Ayizan, a Haitian goddess. Ayizan is parent and protectress to humankind, who keeps us well and safeguards us from malevolent magic. She also teaches us how to effectively make and utilize new things, like technology, in earth-friendly, spiritually fulfilling ways.

MICROWAVE HASTING:

Anytime you need your magic to work quickly, use your microwave to energize it. Find a token that represents the goal of your magic and that can be safely put into the microwave for a few seconds. Put the token in the center of the machine, turn it on for a personally lucky number of seconds (or multiple thereof), and say,

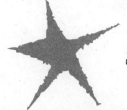

Magic be quick,
move swiftly to tasks.

> When I say the word _____,
> do as I ask.

Remove the token and keep it with you. Whenever you think of it, speak the command word you've chosen while touching your token to activate and motivate the magic toward manifestation.

BLENDER ABUNDANCE:

A blender is the perfect tool for mixing up magic into a harmonious amalgam for just about any need. It can be used to make blends that are consumable or blends of magical ingredients to be used only for symbolic purposes. For example, take some garlic, onion juice, hot sauce, and other "caustic" ingredients, along with any small bell (these are easy to find at craft shops). Put the herbs and juices in the blender, and while it whips the components, say,

> Where this liquid abides,
> no evil may dwell.
> Ayizan stand by my side,
> when thrice rings this bell.

Ring the bell three times.

Next, pour all but a little bit of the mixture into a glass jar and bury it somewhere on the property. The heat of the mixture will repel negativity. Put the remaining liquid in a small unbreakable container that you can keep in the car, a briefcase, or wherever you feel the need.

To change the purpose of this spell, try using different settings on the blender to accent different energy. Use "puree" to get minute details on a situation, "chop" to break up negativity, "dice" to dispel a dicey situation, and "liquefy" to smooth things over!

LOVIN' IN THE OVEN:

Feeling like your love life could use a little heating up? Use your oven to help (even a toaster oven will do)! Begin with a batch of cookies or a slice of sweet bread, which represent sweetness and pleasure. As you bake either, keep an image of your partner in mind. Whisper this phrase: *"Passion, warm, in our hearts be born."* Wrap the cookies or bread in erotic red paper, deliver them to your partner, along with yourself, and enjoy!

To keep the energy of passion and romance active no matter where you may be, simply let one of the cookies or bread get hard and stale, and shellac it so you can carry it.

CHILL OUT!

Everyone has moments of anger. This little bit of magic cools over-heated tempers and opens the way for positive communication. Find or make an emblem of the situation in which emotions need to be cooled off or of the person you're angry at. Put it in the refrigerator. Each time you open the door and see the emblem say, *"Keep the peace, hostility cease."* Begin making efforts toward rectification, and continue using the incantation when you open the refrigerator until things improve. At this point you can take the emblem out and carry it with you to help you keep a cool head even during the most hectic of days. To invoke the magic, just repeat the incantation again (or something similar to it).

FREEZE FRAME:

When you need to stop a problem without directly interfering, this is a terrific spell. It also works very neatly for halting gossip or undesired affections. Simply write the circumstances on a piece of paper. Burn the paper and retain the ashes. Put the ashes in a freezer tray with water, and literally freeze the negativity, gossip, or infatuation. Keep these ice cubes tucked in the back of the freezer until you feel the problem is completely resolved, then let them melt in a garden so that good things grow out of that situation.

If you need to transport the magic, just use a little cooler and some Blue Ice to keep everything frozen.

FLASH OF INSIGHT:

When you want a little inspiration or an improved perspective, use your camera to help. For this spell, close your eyes and relax, keeping your camera in hand and ready to use. Visualize the creative energy of the universe filling you from above and flowing down to your hands. When your hands feel warm, randomly snap some pictures. Have these developed and look to see what images form. For example, if you needed perspective about a love affair and the camera captured a burning fire, this means your relationship has gotten too hot.

If you are using the spell for ideas, carry the photographs with you. Hold them in your hand whenever you need extra inventiveness, and let the energy of the visualization fill you again. Then, set about your tasks!

VCR VERIFICATION:

Feeling uncertain about something? Get an answer from your VCR! While thinking about a specific question, randomly choose any movie and put it in the player. Fast-forward the movie, again keeping your question in mind, and repeat three times, *"Pictures that move, pictures that fly, bring to me a true reply."* Stop the movie and listen to the first phrase spoken, and write it down. This will somehow answer your question. The paper acts as a portable charm to enable effective action.

Alternative Components:

Use yellow highlights for the conscious mind (perhaps yellow lined paper), jet pieces (a stone) near any "technological" items to help keep them working well, quartz for general energy and creativity, and spearmint or rosemary incense for mental keenness. Try using doorbells or telephones in spells for receiving news, chant magical missives through household intercoms, use pilot lights as a fire emblem, faucets for water, air conditioners for air, and the cellar floor for earth.

The timing for techno-magic depends heavily on the need at hand. Consider the first signs of a crescent moon for fresh beginnings, Tuesdays to accentuate skill and logic, the month of June for composure and good decision making, and when the moon is in Sagittarius for improved will power.

Around the House

As you can see, the trend in this book is to appreciate the magic in everything, including all the corners of your living space. If you never thought of the bathroom as magical, for example, just turn the lock and sit down with a good book—this is a perfect "spell" for privacy!

For magic in any part of the house, call on Kikimora, the Slavonic domestic goddess. She is an especially good choice for those of us who feel domestically challenged. As an offering to grab her attention, wash a pot or pan in fern tea before beginning your magic. Or, more simply, attach a dried fern frond to a decorative pot that you hang in the kitchen or your sacred space.

SELF-BLESSING SHOWER:

Few of us take enough time in self-blessings. A moment to bless yourself is the most important time of any day. It attracts the Goddess's energy and assistance to you, and it will help any magic you may create. For the blessing shower, begin with fragrant herbs like lavender flowers for peace, catnip leaves for attractiveness, allspice beads for health and luck, and a cinnamon stick for love and power. Bundle these in loosely woven cloth or soft netting. As you wash, gently rub this all over your body to clean away negativity, saying,

> Cares wash away;
> keep misfortune at bay.
> Kikimora touch me,
> your blessings I'll see!

As you do this, imagine the water appearing like sparkling silver light that absorbs any troubles, then washes away.

Afterward, take a smaller bundle of the herbs with you to keep the blessings and protective energies activated.

FLUSH YOUR TROUBLES AWAY:

The next time you're enjoying a moment of privacy on the proverbial "throne," take the opportunity to weave a little magic. Using the symbolism of flushing as central to your spell, you can use any handy stall to flush away a source of trouble! Just draw an image of the difficulty on a piece of toilet paper and toss it in! When you flush, don't look at the paper—just turn away, so you don't figuratively accept the problem back.

DUST BUSTER EXORCISM:

Think your house is haunted, or perhaps the walls are just screaming with too much irritation? Unvex it with a hex! Take some salt and sprinkle it counterclockwise around the inside perimeter of your living space, repeating this phrase purposefully as you go: *"Away from me, spirits and negativity."* Next, take a hand vacuum and clean up the salt clockwise, saying, *"Magic, shine. This space is mine!"*

If you're someplace where a hand vacuum isn't available, like a hotel room or bed-and-breakfast, you can sweep up the salt using a piece of paper or your hand instead.

LIGHTEN UP!

Sometimes it seems as if the universe were dumping all over our reality. It's pretty tough to keep our spirits bright during these disastrous days, but some scented oils and a few lamps can help. Choose an oil that is directly opposite to your mood. For example, if you're angry, get apple blossom for joy. If you're sick, use violet or rosemary for health, and if besieged by rotten luck, use cinnamon, clove, or vanilla oil. Whatever your choice, dab this on every lamp you come in contact with. That way, whenever you need a lift, you can literally lighten up just by switching on the lamp.

DO IT BY THE NUMBERS:

This is a type of divination that you can use anywhere. Think of your question, visualizing it in as much detail as possible with your eyes closed. After opening your eyes, write down the first number you see on any object (like the numbers on a clock or in a ZIP code on a letter, the weight measurement on canned goods, etc.). If the number is larger than 10, add the digits together so you can get a single-digit response. For example, if you see the ZIP code 14224, add $1+4+2+2+4 = 13 = 1+3 = 4$. This number represents the response to your question, as follows:

1 = You probably have to go this alone. Let your ambition and drive act as a companion.

2 = Use diplomacy and sensitivity to sort this out.

3 = Be more flexible and tolerant.

4 = Think logically about this question, and the answer will make itself known.

5 = No matter what the question, adventure is on the horizon.

6 = Romance or new friendships are developing.

7 = Your intuition knows best and will bring you luck. You might want to play this number in the lottery!

8 = Some type of rebound or recuperation is coming.

9 = A fight is imminent, either with another person or in the form of a struggle to assert personal ideals.

When using this as a portable technique, just change your focus to suit the circumstance. Look at license plates, bulletin boards, exit numbers, and the like for the numerical response.

BOOGIE FEVER:

Music soothes the savage beast, so why not use it magically to soothe the soul? For this spell, I suggest calling on Bast instead of Kikimora, since Bast is the goddess of dance, joy, and playfulness. Find a piece of music that makes you feel like dancing. Play it loudly, and begin dancing clockwise around your living space. As you dance, sing or chant to the music. Add a rhythmic incantation like *"The joy of dance, prance with me! By Bast's power, joy be free!"* Start this incantation quietly and let it naturally increase with the pace of your dance. When you feel the energy reach a pinnacle, raise your hands on the word *free* to release the magic of happiness into your home.

Alternative Components:

For this spell you can use components as diverse and varied as is your living space. Look around your home with a different perspective to see the magical potential there. For example, consider drawing heavy curtains to shut out negativity or improve privacy. Open your windows and let the winds of change do their work. Or, use a mirror and cleaning solution as an alternative scrying surface!

Time household magic according to what your schedule will allow. Friday nights are one good choice, since Friday is the end of the average work week and a day that accentuates good relationships and effective communication. Any day in the month of August improves harmony, and working when the moon is in Aquarius cultivates empathy.

PC and Internet Incantations

These days you can do just about everything with a home computer or on the Internet, so why not a little magic? Think of electricity as the power, and the networks or file functions as the guiding lines, and you begin to see how your magical energy can travel where it's most needed. For example, if you're submitting a resume to a company, or sending a message to which you want to attach a little purposeful magic, recite this phrase while preparing and sending the document:

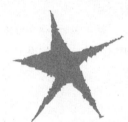

Computer network,
guide well this spark,
through bits and bytes
to hit my mark.

Accent this spell by burning symbolic incense as you work. Relight the incense anytime to support the magic.

There are two goddesses suited to computer and Internet magic. The first is Vach, the Hindu goddess of mystic speech through which wisdom is imparted. Her help can apply to any programming difficulties or Internet file forwarding. The second is Tashmit, the Chaldean goddess of hearing and speech who makes those receiving messages more open to their content. She is an excellent choice for blessing and empowering your e-mail.

FILE IT!
What do you need in your life right now? Think about it, and find a short word that describes that need. Then create a special file on your computer that details mundane efforts you can make to meet that need. Name the file with the short word you chose, like *victory, health,* or *money.* Then each time you access that computer file, you will literally retrieve into your life the magical energy of victory, health, money, or whatever you chose, while continuing conventional efforts toward that end!

For those of you without computers, or who want a more portable spell, use file folders instead. These fit neatly into suitcases and briefcases for similar ends.

A LUCKY MOUSE IN THE HOUSE.
In Eastern lands, people often keep a cricket found in their home in a special cage to bring luck, and in Bohemia white mice are considered very fortunate. Putting these two ideas together, keep your computer mouse in special housing (computer stores sell these) when it's not in use. In the bottom of whatever storage area you choose, place something that represents an area in which you need more luck—for example, use a heart-shaped piece of paper for love, or a coin covered in green cloth for prosperity.

Keep the symbol stored there for a personally lucky number of days or weeks, so your little white mouse can infuse it with lucky energy. Every time you see it say,

> *Little mouse inside your cage,*
> *with lucky energy this token pervade.*
> *Tashmit my wish shall transmit,*
> *each time these buttons get hit.*

Carry the symbol with you, and repeat the incantation each time you use your mouse, until the magic manifests.

SCREEN SAVER SAVVY:
Another good way to help manifest your magic is to support it through imagery that you see regularly. Look through different screen savers and find one that best represents your magical goal. Try to create an incantation that you recite each time this image comes on your screen. This motivates magical energy to support any spells you're currently working on.

THE FISHING LINE:
A lot of folks go surfing the Internet to find other people of a like mind, hoping to make long-distance friends. This spell helps achieve that goal.

To begin, get a three-foot length of fishing line (or any thread) and take it to where you work on your computer. Write the word *friend* on a piece of paper and tie it to one end of the fishing line. Place that end of the line across the computer desk from you and the other end in your hand. Make sure your computer is booted up to whatever network you use for chatting with people. Now, focus on your intention, and slowly draw the string into your hand, saying, *"Friends to find, for friends I fish, through this line, to Vach I send my wish!"* Keep repeating this phrase until the paper is in your hand. Wrap it with the length of fishing line and have it with you each time you access the Internet looking for companions.

Alternative Components:

Pale yellow accents effective communication. Keep amethyst near gadgets so you don't lose your cool when working with them. Use typing stands and clipboards to hold magical emblems, neatly binding the magic to that area. Bad computer disks or CDs can be cleansed, blessed, and empowered for a specific function, then used as energetic coasters. And, put a positive password on your computer so each time you open a program, you "open" that energy!

Good times for computer and Internet magic (besides whenever things don't seem to be working) include noontime and Sundays, when the sun's logical influence can help the most; the month of March for mastery, or September to understand "mysterious" things, and when the moon is in Libra, for sound judgment.

Pampered Pets

For many people, their pets are like children to pamper and protect. Pocket magic meets this need by suggesting charms, special bedding, and rituals that guard the creature against sickness and misfortune.

The perfect goddess to help with pet magic is Brigit. She is an Irish deity who protects animals and presides over all household arts. As the daughter of the good god Dagda, she was renowned for her acts of gentleness and kindness to all creatures.

FRISKY ELDER FLOWERS:

English folklore tells us that elder flowers protect animals. To activate this magic and make an effective flea-deterrent bed, mingle dried elder flowers in cedar shavings and sew them into a large pillow for your pet. If you happen to have fish or birds, I suggest keeping dried elder flowers attached to the bowl or cage instead. As you work on the bed, invoke Brigit's blessing, saying,

> Brigit abide by my pet's side.
> Keep _____ safe and well,
> let your magic here always dwell.

Make a smaller, sachet-sized token, so you can keep it with your pet no matter where you may be.

"DOG" TAG CHARMS:

For cats and dogs, this bit of magic requires either an ID tag or a bell. For birds, use a slightly larger bell; for fish, use a submergible token. Take whatever object you've chosen and hold it in your hand. Visualize bright, white, protective light filling the charm as you say,

Health, long life, befall no harm,
all while you wear this magic charm.

Put this on you pet's collar, or wherever they will be around the item regularly. Recharge the object from time to time to keep the magic fully activated.

A MOMENT'S PAWS:

Another bit of folklore says that buttering an animal's paws will keep it from ever getting lost. I suggest using shortening instead, which is also good for preventing hair balls should the animal lick the substance off. Take a small amount of shortening and warm it with garlic for protection, then let it cool. Dab this on your pet's paws once a month, saying,

One for love,
two for a long life wherever you roam,
three for health,
four that you may ne'er stray from home.

THE BRUSH-OFF:

Want to keep your animals free from fleas and protect them, too? This is the perfect spell. Take four cups of water and add eight drops each of rosemary, sage, cedar, and fennel oil (all of which deter fleas and have magical protective qualities). Stir these counter-clockwise during a waning or dark moon, saying, *"Pests be gone, go forever away! All fleas and maladies be kept at bay."* Brush this into the creature's hair once a week. Also, dip your pet's collar in the mixture and let it dry, then put the collar back on the animal so your magic and love will always be with them.

Alternative Components:

Rich browns or greens accent nature's power. Fill your pet's dishes with specially prepared foods or crystal tinctures. Place a blessed, charged moonstone in the area where the creature spends most of its time, for restful sleep. Use charmed valerian or catnip for cats and an enchanted bone for dogs.

Good times for making these charms or performing spells are Saturday, which is named after Saturn, who presides over natural cycles; during the month of May, which is named after the goddess Maia, an earth deity; and when the moon is in any earth sign (Capricorn, Virgo, Taurus).

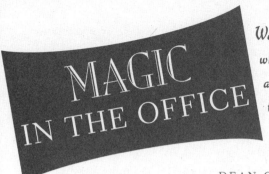

We have too many people who live without working, and we have altogether too many who work without living!

—DEAN CHARLES R. BROWN

When you get up and go to work each day, your spirit travels with you as a figurative backseat driver. It guides the interactions you have with people and how you handle difficult situations. So, when you leave the house, don't leave behind the Goddess and her magic. Tuck it in your pocket, then find creative ways to release her power into your job.

Start your day by dusting your shoes with dynamic, charismatic herbs like cinnamon. Or, consider wearing clothing whose colors accent successful characteristics for your job. A supervisor, for instance, might wear yellow-reds to motivate creative leadership qualities; a nurse might don purple, a color that engenders sympathy, and a writer might wear yellow for creativity. Perfumes and colognes also work wonders. Simply dab on some symbolic aromatics first thing in the morning. Here the supervisor might add pennyroyal oil for productivity, and the nurse would choose geranium oil to protect his or her health.

Decorate your work space for optimum power. Keep magically charged crystals nearby (see chapter 1) to give you an extra boost when you most need it. I also find that live plants, if allowed, are very useful. You can pick the plant according to its powers, but any growing plant symbolizes the manifestation of your desires.

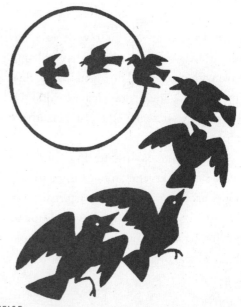

Machinery Magic

Who couldn't use a little magic around our beloved, can't-live-with-out-'em office machines? As we become more dependent on technology, our need for magic and spirituality also increases. When you experience answering machine failure, computer crashes, or cranky photocopiers, you can always call a repair person, but why not also try a little magic? Magic, being of an electrical nature, works marvelously with most technological gadgets. If nothing else, it gives you something productive to do while you wait for help!

For goddesses turn to Tara, the Indian goddess of knowledge, control, and good judgment. Tara rides a lion, with the sun of understanding in one hand, to save the creatures of the world from all terrors, including those caused by impatient bosses! Alternatively, consider Danu, the Irish patroness of sorcerers and wizards (today's technology being yesterday's magic). Invoke Danu by carrying barley in your pocket as you work.

R & R (REPAIR & RESTORATION):

To speed along computer repairs, burn a stick of rosemary incense in the area where you're working (or dab some rosemary oil on yourself). The entire time you (or a repair person) work on the machine, mentally recite,

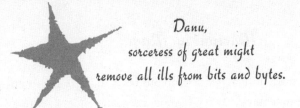

Danu,
sorceress of great might
remove all ills from bits and bytes.

The repairs should be completed properly by the time the rosemary burns out.

For a portable charm, keep a small amount of the rosemary ashes and put them in a breakproof container. Sprinkle these in any region where you need improved mental focus.

COPIER CONCESSIONS:

During a waning moon, take an offering of toner to your copier. While you replace this and clean out the component parts, ask for Tara's blessing. Leave a bay leaf under each wheel of the machine to keep it safeguarded against future problems.

Bay leaves make an excellent pocket charm for continued strength, protection, and overall energy while at the office. Write the word *energy* on the leaf and keep it tucked in your wallet or shoe.

TELEPHONE TAG:

Place the image of an open hand under your telephone when lines are busy or down to help you "reach out and touch someone." After the lines clear, toss the image into the trash so it will carry troubles away from the phone.

Draw the same image on another piece of paper, saying,

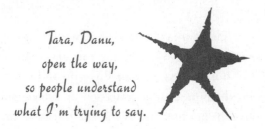

Tara, Danu,
open the way,
so people understand
what I'm trying to say.

Carry this image in your purse, wallet, briefcase, or pocket to improve your communications throughout the office (or anywhere else, for that matter).

HUM-ALONG HEALING:

I have a friend who swears by this method. When any machine is giving you trouble, begin to hum or "tone" to it. Use low, even sounds, as close as possible to any it makes. Focus your mind on the vibrations of that sound, and on how it makes you feel. This will slowly bring you into harmony with the machine, which will result in one of two things: either the machine will start working better, or you will suddenly realize what you're doing wrong.

The nice part about this method is that your voice is a perfectly portable component for pocket magic. Getting impatient for an elevator, for example? Start humming!

JUST THE FAX:

If you find your fax (or modem) always hangs up mid-transmission, use a little magic to smooth the lines of communication. Put a dab of coffee (for energy) on your fingertip and trace a banishing pentagram three times (for protection and alleviating troubles) on the side of the machine (begin and end tracing at the lower left point of the star). As you sketch, visualize white light being absorbed by the machine and traveling through the electrical connections to open them.

This spell can be used anywhere—just change the anointing liquid to suit the circumstances and availability. For example, dab on water to improve figurative flow, tea to encourage tranquillity, or orange juice to restore "health."

Alternative Components:

Use orange peel or oil to help divine the problem and envision positive solutions, and mint extract to exorcise bad spirits from the machine. Hematite stones near the work area ground out electrical troubles, a fossil will help keep the item working longer, and jet or tiger's eye will bring luck.

Keep foods and beverages out of this kind of magic—crumbs and liquids have a very bad karmic effect on anything electrical. And, by all means, don't forget to bless your tool kit and instruction manuals, perhaps dabbing a little rosemary oil on them to improve reasoning abilities.

For timing, consider a waning moon or new moon for banishing the machine's demons; when the moon is in Taurus for common sense; the month of July to keep from losing your cool; Sunday to accent reason, or Saturday to effect an outcome.

Managing Your Manager

Do you feel like your manager doesn't hear what you're saying, doesn't seem to appreciate your efforts, or doesn't give you due credit? Do you just need to communicate with this person in a more positive, self-assured manner? A little office magic can really help. These sample charms and spells open the door for improving your relationship with any authority figure, and they also aid in regaining control in that environment.

For manager magic, turn to Athena, the Greek goddess of warriors and commerce. Athena protected common workers like craftspeople, weavers, and smiths. Mythology also portrays her as being a source of good advice, peace, and justice, and as inspiring effective strategy. Honor her in the sacred space with handcrafted items, flute music, olives, and musk incense.

GOOD, GOOD, GOOD, VIBRATIONS:

To promote peaceful vibrations in and around the work space, grow lavender at your desk. Adding stones to the soil will further accentuate the energies. For example, put a red agate in the southern portion of the planter for bold action, a white agate in the east for inner peace, a brown agate in the north for resourcefulness, and a green agate in the west for growing self-assurance.

Keep matching stones for yourself. Empower them by saying,

Athena, fill these stones with peace and action bold,
when I take them in my hand, let the magic unfold.
Fill them with poise and attentiveness,
that where'er I go I shall be blessed.

Carry these in a medicine pouch or other bundle to keep their positive energy with you everywhere.

PEACE IS PERKING:

If your manager drinks tea, make him or her a special blend that includes some dried violet for harmony. Alternatively, look at the supermarket for chamomile tea (another herb that inspires peace). Sweeten it to sweeten your manager's disposition.

For coffee lovers, make a tea out of any symbolic (edible) herb, and keep it refrigerated until needed. Add a few drops to the coffee. The amount doesn't matter; the vibrations of the herbs themselves do the trick. Stir clockwise for positive, empowering energy, or counterclockwise to decrease negativity.

OFFERING THE OLIVE BRANCH:

Draw a peace symbol on an olive leaf, or on any white paper. Over this, visualize your boss's image. Dab a little White Out on the leaf as you visualize, to figuratively erase the problems. Fold it inward thrice (the number of body-mind-spirit in balance), wrapping it around a small malachite as you fold (the stone is optional). Carry this in your wallet or keep it in your desk until things improve. Then burn the paper while giving thanks, and keep the stone nearby so it continues to promote positive interactions.

APPRECIATION AMULET:

When you want your supervisor to notice your efforts more, try making this amulet for yourself. Begin with a slice of pine wood. Using indelible marker or paint, draw the rune *Dagaz* on the slice (this looks like two sideways triangles with their tips touching). *Dagaz* represents achievements and opportunity and can be considered the "carpe diem" of runes. As you draw the rune, say,

Let worthy work receive due praise
as I toil, long, hard days.
Let my skills and talents shine
whene'er I wear this charm of pine.

If you feel uncomfortable wearing this on a necklace, simply punch a hole in it and attach it to your key chain instead.

MOOD MAGIC:

Has your supervisor been grumpy, discontented, or out of sorts? Is this making *everyone* miserable? Try a little aro-magical assistance! At home, prepare a tea from one cup of water, one apple-flavored tea bag (for happiness), one Earl Grey tea bag (to turn negativity), a pinch of rosemary (for healing), and a pinch of basil (for harmony). Stir the mixture counterclockwise, saying, *"Unhappiness fade, discontent cease."* Then stir clockwise, saying, *"Rediscover peace, with each breath, joy's released!"* Let this steep until it has a heady scent. Store it in a dark, airtight container in the refrigerator until you have a chance to apply it to areas where your manager spends a lot of his or her time.

Alternative Components:

Put apples or peaches in your lunch for discernment, or alternatively bring in apple fritters for healthy discourse. Wear yellow for creative communication. Keep malachite with you for improved business success or an agate for courage.

Time your efforts by a waxing moon to improve discourse, or a waning moon to decrease negativity. Spells and charms enacted on Thursday help maintain tenacity and meet obligations. The month of January is good for protection, while March overcomes difficulty, and April creates opportunities. Working when the moon is in Libra will ensure you receive fair treatment.

Preventing Office Politics

No matter where we work, few of us are completely free from office politics or the ever-grinding rumor mill. Either situation can make getting ready for work dreadful. So, to fill your mornings with anticipation instead of trepidation, whip up a little magic and astrally kick some bureaucratic butt!

Turn to Sin, the Teutonic goddess of truth, for help in such matters, or alternatively, to Ma'at, the Egyptian goddess of justice and universal law. This way, even if you have to endure periodic office politics, the results will be equitable.

THE TERMINATION TALISMAN:

When you've grown weary of people who need to "get a life" instead of nosing into yours, make a protective talisman to turn their attentions elsewhere. You need a sharp pin and a small mirror, like those in compacts, or any highly polished surface, like that of a metallic pen. The shiny surface reflects away unwanted energy.

Work during a waning moon so that your problems will shrink into nothingness. Take the shiny surface and scratch the rune of protection (this looks like a Y with the middle line slightly extended upward) into it, saying,

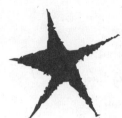

Away from me, negativity.
Unwanted attention shall fade.
Gossip and politics cannot abide
where'er this talisman lies.

Hide the talisman in a safe spot where people most often shoot the breeze or where you feel the greatest source of trouble stews. If you want some pocket magic to accompany this effort, simply make two talismans at the same time and keep one with you.

DISTRACTION TACTICS:

Sometimes the greatest way to keep people from getting you involved in unwanted group dynamics is to divert attentions elsewhere. For this spell, you'll need a bit of your personally favored cologne or perfume and an old key. Dab the chosen scent lightly around the area in which you work. As you do, visualize bands of white light connecting each dot of aromatic to the others. Similar to the way animals mark their territory, this symbolically and metaphysically marks your personal territory and issues a powerful challenge to any daring to enter without being welcome.

Second, take the key and dab it with four drops of the scent. As you do, try an incantation like this one:

On the count of four, I close the door.
On the count of three, stay away from me.
On the count of two, let Sin's magic ring true.
On the count of one, this spell's begun.

Keep this charm in your desk, a locker, or your pocket. Anytime you feel that someone is trying to draw you into unproductive political banter, turn the key in your pocket to turn attention elsewhere.

RUMOR ROUSTER:

When the rumor mill starts working "24–7" there comes a time when enough is enough. If you've reached your limit of unproductive, misleading, and sometimes hurtful conversations, zap them with magic. Take a pencil, pen, or anything that can become a pointer and aim the tip toward the source of trouble. Mentally recite this invocation seven times:

Ma'at, make the mayhem cease.
Let the truth be released.

As you repeat the phrase, visualize beams of light being emitting from the tip and piercing the troublemaker(s) through the heart. This acts as a mystical moralistic nudge directed to the person's ethical center.

ARMISTICE AMULET:

Want the tensions and hostilities in your office to cease? A peaceful amulet may be just the what the safety officer ordered. Begin with an all-white piece of paper, which represents a flag of truce. Draw an image of the peace symbol on the paper using some personal cologne or perfume. This represents your willingness to work toward restitution. Fold the image three times in toward itself, saying,

> *Let peace be born in place of ire.*
> *I release this prayer to the cleansing fire.*

Burn the paper in a fire-safe container, then carry the ashes with you until the situation resolves. Afterward, release the ashes to the winds as a way of sharing peace with the planet.

POLITICAL SAVVY:

Sometimes there's no avoiding office politics. When this happens, use a little magic to make yourself as effective as possible. For this spell I've used consumable charms, so you will literally internalize

the energy and carry it with you through the day. If possible, prepare this meal when the moon is in Aries, which accentuates leadership abilities and courage.

Before going to work, make yourself an empowering meal.
Have grape juice to strengthen mental abilities, some ginger-and-
cinnamon-dusted toast for power, blackberries for protection, and a
glass of milk, which represents the Goddess. Say a brief prayer over
these to invite the Goddess's blessing. Eat expectantly!

Alternative Components:

A stack of interoffice memo paper scented with lavender, rose,
or violet will promote peaceful communications. Add any knickknacks with blue coloring to the office to accent harmony. Bless and
empower doughnuts for sweet discourse.

For timing, consider a dark moon to end problems cleanly and
let them die. Working on a Friday improves relationships of all
types, the month of August accentuates agreement and unity, and
an Aquarius moon augments benevolence.

Efficiency Enchantments

Efficiency is something all of us can use, no matter where we may be. It helps get everything done quickly so there's time left for fun and relaxation! At our jobs, being competent and productive makes the day run smoothly, with fewer crises and less stress. For all those workaholics out there, this also means fewer anxiety attacks!

For matters requiring orderliness, call on Eunomia, the Greek goddess of organization (the daughter of Zeus and faithful attendant to Hera), to keep you on track.

WHISTLE WHILE YOU WORK:

Don't underestimate the power of music as both a universal language and a medium for the Goddess's energy. Find a few songs that make you feel upbeat, good about yourself, and motivated. Memorize at least one verse of each. Then, each time you start feeling unable to cope or really wiped out at work, hum or whistle a happy tune. For example, popular New Age songs like *Tallis the Messenger* (David Arkenstone), classics like *Carmina burana,* and magically focused songs like *All Soul's Night* (Loreena McKennitt) all help me direct my efforts more effectively and joyfully.

Once known, this magical music will always be with you, making it the perfect magic to pull out of your pocket for a little extra energy anytime!

ORGANIZATION OGHAM:

Oghams are an ancient form of writing from the Celtic tradition, each symbol of which represents a tree with specific meaning. The Oghams were required learning for druids, necessary to obtaining mastery, which is the perfect symbolism for methodical magic! In this case, you will be using the symbol for apple, which consists of one vertical line with five small horizontal lines attached at equal intervals on the left side of the vertical one. Apple represents personal mastery that results in no wasted energy.

Begin by slicing an apple across the center so that the pentagram formed by the seeds can be seen. Make another cut so you have a one-fourth-inch-by-one-half-inch slice showing this natural magical star. Using a toothpick, carve the apple Ogham into the slice at the four compass points, repeating this invocation at each point:

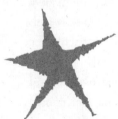

Powers of the North and East,
obey my will, make bedlam cease!
Powers of the South and West,
Eunomia, help me do my best!

Keep this in an arid, cool area until it dries completely, and then shellac it. Carry it with you whenever you need to come up with better strategies. If you leave a hole at the top of this amulet you can wear it on a necklace, hang it in a window, or even make several with different symbols for Yule decorations!

CAPABILITY CHARM:

Find any square object that you can keep near yourself at work. Examples include a square mouse pad, a pencil or paper clip holder, or a belt buckle. The square symbolizes orderliness and strong foundations. Take this in hand at noon to accentuate logic and progress. Visualize the golden sunlight filling it as you say,

Golden rays of sun, divine,
through me let competence and proficiency shine.

If you want to make a portable charm at the same time, find a squarish stone and empower it similarly.

PRODUCTIVITY POWER:

During the time of a waxing moon, take a two-liter bottle of ginger ale (for effervescent energy), add one clove bud (for good judgment), a teaspoon of coconut flavoring (for flexibility), and a twist of lemon (for clarity). Close this up tightly and hold it upward toward the sky, saying,

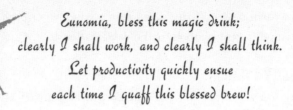

Eunomia, bless this magic drink;
clearly I shall work, and clearly I shall think.
Let productivity quickly ensue
each time I quaff this blessed brew!

Drink a little sip before you set about your tasks to carry the power with you. You can also bundle up an extra clove bud, a bit of coconut, and a dry lemon rind in a sachet and dab it with the ginger ale. Leave this in your car, a suitcase, a briefcase, or wherever you feel it's needed.

Alternative Components:

Anoint memo pads or bulletin boards on which you can keep a "to do" list. Engrave on the back of your watch a magical emblem like the rune *Raido* to keep you prompt (this rune looks like an R in which the curve of the letter is pointed, and it represents juggling multiple elements successfully). Use anything with a rich, brown color, which represents good foundations. Crystals like bloodstone and malachite will help to achieve business success.

Time your efforts to coincide with a full moon for completion. Enact them on Tuesdays for increased skill, during the month of July for self-control, or when the moon is in Virgo for practicality.

Promotion Potions

Haven't had a review lately? Wish that your administrators appreciated your skills more? Tired of living off macaroni and cheese? If you're long overdue for a raise or promotion at work, it's time to return to your cauldron of ideas and whip up some creative magic.

To help with advancement magic, call on the Roman goddess Fortuna, who oversees all matters of fate and fortune. Her color is gold, and her symbol is a wheel. This might translate into carrying a gold-colored coin or wearing a gold ring to invoke Fortuna's positive attentions.

LET'S DO LUNCH:

A week before your review, or before asking for a raise, start eating your way to prosperity. To accomplish this, include in your lunches foods and beverages whose energies encourage abundance—for instance, any berry-flavored waters (representing earth's bounty), green or leafy foods like broccoli and lettuce (representing the color and texture of money), and gourmet goodies (which are usually treats reserved for times when we have extra money). Pray before you eat, stating your needs to Fortuna, or use this invocation:

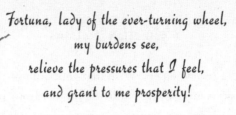

> *Fortuna, lady of the ever-turning wheel,*
> *my burdens see,*
> *relieve the pressures that I feel,*
> *and grant to me prosperity!*

Accent this magic by wearing green garments daily (don't forget that socks and underwear count), and wearing vetiver oil, which draws riches and motivates positive change.

ADVANCEMENT AMULET:

Concerned that your hours might be cut, that a demotion is imminent, or that downsizing is around the corner? Make this amulet to protect yourself from these kinds of changes; you might even improve your status through proactive magic.

Begin working on the last night of the full moon. Take a small item that somehow represents your position and a white cloth, and set them in the moonlight. This charges the token so that it provides you with mature insights. On the next night, take the cloth and token in hand beneath the moon, saying,

> *Misfortune, stay away from me;*
> *only prosperity shall I see.*

Keep my job safe from all harm.
Fortuna, empower this magic charm.

Wrap the token in the cloth and carry it with you, or keep it where you spend the most time at work.

This charm can be changed to meet a lot of different needs. For example, if you've been having a period of bad luck, just find an object that represents fortuity to you, and rewrite the invocation to something like the following:

Misfortune, stay away from me;
Only good luck shall I see.
Fortuna, infuse this charm with serendipity!

FORTUNE FETISH:

To make a fortune fetish, begin with a round tie tack or pin that has a green stone set in it, or one that is made from gold-colored metal. The circular shape symbolizes Fortuna, while green and gold vibrate with prosperous energy. If possible, prepare the fetish just before midnight, during a waxing moon in the month of April to emphasize a change toward improved fortunes.

Take the chosen token and cup it in both hands. Begin to chant quietly, with your eyes closed,

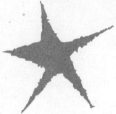

> Prosperity, luck, and Fortuna's power,
> fill this token
> come the witching hour.

Let the volume of this chant rise naturally with the chiming of midnight, and stop with the last bell. Wear this any time you feel you need a little extra money or luck.

CLIMBING THE CORPORATE LADDER:

If you have stairs at your office, or anywhere nearby, this little bit of sympathetic magic will help you improve your business prospects. Each time you go up any set of stairs, mentally recite an incantation like this one:

> As I climb,
> fortune is mine!
> Up I go, beyond all foes.
> Prosperity and fame,
> success I claim!

The movement up the stairs symbolizes ascent, thereby supporting your magical focus. You can use this type of sympathetic magic for overcoming problems. Or reverse the process when you go down the stairs, for goals having to do with releasing negativity or the past.

ENRICHMENT ELIXIR:

Looking for a bolstering brew? Begin with any juice that you enjoy. Magically, juice accents well-being, physical health, and happiness. Add to this a little productive visualization, seeing the entire container filled with the golden light of the sun, which symbolizes the Goddess's blessing. Then, hold the pitcher in hand, and recite a prayer/incantation like this one:

Through the teeth, past the gums,
throughout my body, wellness comes.
When this touches to my lips
abundance dwells inside each sip!

Pour yourself a glass each morning and each night, repeating your incantation before quaffing your magic.

Alternative Components:

For raises, coins and dollar bills figure heavily into prosperity magic. For example, turn a silver coin in your pocket when you first see a new moon to draw more money to you. Write your wish for abundance on a dollar and burn this mixed with dried oak leaves. The smoke will carry your wish to the Goddess and release the energy of abundance. Or, bless your wallet or money clip so it attracts cash.

For timing, consider working during the full moon, which represents both plenty and completion, on a Saturday to reap the harvest of hard labor, during the month of October for positive change, or when the moon is in Taurus for abundance.

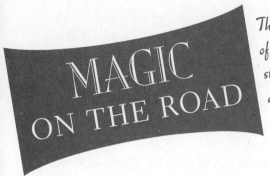

MAGIC ON THE ROAD

The world is a great book, of which they who never stir from home read only a page.

—ST. AUGUSTINE

How often have you arrived at a destination late or frazzled because of problems along the way? Ever had reservations get completely messed up, or received incorrect directions? In a mobile society, portable magic becomes all the more important and useful. Whether you commute two miles or two hundred, taking the Goddess along bypasses many problems.

Put an amulet in your attaché case, hang a talisman in your car's trunk, make a fetish for your foot locker and an enchanted sachet for your suitcase. From the moment you head out the door, for whatever reason, hold tight to the Goddess and her magic, especially when the ride gets bumpy. She can keep you safer and far less aggravated, whatever the mode of transportation!

Travel Talismans

Consider this section a magical Triple-A. When you're traveling, the Goddess's energy remains at home to keep it safe, but it can also travel with you in simple ways. Don't be deceived by a spell or charm's simplicity—just because something's uncomplicated doesn't mean it lacks power. In fact, keeping traveling magic simple gives you more time to direct the energy you create, and more time to have fun!

For goddesses, consider Artemis, to whom Greek travelers turned when they wanted pleasant weather, or Hina, the Polynesian patroness of travelers. Artemis can be invoked with acorns, and Hina can be honored with any two-sided item.

X MARKS THE SPOT:

If you ever have the chance to go anywhere you want without tons of preplanning, dousing offers one way to find magical getaway spots. Find a Y-shaped branch, preferably of hazel, willow, apple, or maple, and get out a map of the surrounding area. Grasp the two short ends of the branch, one in each hand. Stand back from the table so that the tip of the long end of the branch is parallel with the center of the map. Close your eyes and say,

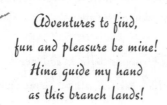

Adventures to find,
fun and pleasure be mine!
Hina guide my hand
as this branch lands!

Allow the branch to tip downward until it touches the map. Open your eyes to reveal your destination!

If you want to find some interesting sites while in your hotel room, where you probably won't have a branch handy, use a pencil instead. Hold the pencil above the map with your eyes closed, and keep moving it clockwise until you finish the incantation. Then put the point down. Where the point lands marks the spot where your adventure begins.

SAFETY FIRST:

One concern people have when on the road is safety. While you might trust your driving, the bus driver's driving, or the pilot's flying, you can't always trust the "other guy." And having your pocket picked, or vacationing during an earthquake, is not most people's idea of a good time.

To magically safeguard yourself, get a small mirror, preferably one that fits nicely in a pocket, a purse, or a camera case. Hold the mirror in your hands and turn it counterclockwise three times, repeating this incantation each time:

Dilemmas deflect; evil avert;
bad luck reflect; all problems divert.

Then turn it clockwise three times, saying,

Artemis, in this mirror shine
so that safety will be mine.

Touch the mirror and repeat the incantation anytime you feel the need.

LIVE LIKE A KING ON A PEASANT'S BUDGET:

Most of us average Joes and Jills can't always afford to really pamper ourselves, even on vacation. But, with a little magically inspired luck, things can happen during your travels that make you feel like a king or queen. You might find some extra cash, have a nicer room open up at the hotel, get a free meal for being customer number one thousand, or have some other unexpected luck.

Get seven Apache tears (stones), or seven small pieces of turquoise and a small bag or other container in which to house them. Let the stones soak up the light of a full moon for seven hours. Afterward, take the stones in your hand, saying,

Luck be quick, luck be kind,
by lucky seven, good luck be mine!

Keep these with you as you travel. Whenever you feel you need a little extra good fortune, toss one in any moving water source or fountain as you make your wish.

AW, NUTS!

If situations come up that lead to frustration and undue tension, try this fetish. You will need a small drawstring bag, preferably one made from natural material like cotton or linen. The best color is white, for protection, but this is optional. Go to a nearby park or field where you can gather thirteen acorns (the number of lunar months in a year). Take these in your hand one at a time to drop them in the bag. As you do, use an incantation that designates each acorn as fulfilling a specific need, like

One, my wish for joy; Two, my wish for smooth sailing;
Three, my wish for relaxation; Four, my wish for comfort;
Five, my wish for quiet;
Six, my wish for good traveling companions;
Seven, my wish for pleasant weather; Eight, my wish
for safety;
Nine, my wish for fun; Ten, my wish for adventure;
Eleven, my wish for good travel connections;
Twelve, my wish for a journey filled with pleasant
memories;
Artemis bless these tokens—when they're planted in the
ground
let magic grow and luck abound!

Change the wishes to suit your circumstances and goals. Carry this with you, but plant only one acorn a month unless an emergency arises.

A good time to create this fetish is either on New Year's (eve or day, although the former is more traditional), so magic will flow through your entire year, or during a waning moon, so troubles will go away.

ALL KEYED UP:

I can't tell you how many times I've stayed at a hotel where either other patrons were noisy or people came to my door accidentally, interrupting a perfectly good dream! To prevent this kind of disturbance, use your Do Not Disturb sign as a spell component.

Put a bit of your cologne or perfume on your index finger and use it to trace a peace symbol on the sign. Keep retracing this emblem while visualizing the entire sign glowing with vibrant white light. When the sign has absorbed all the energy it can (it may feel warm in your hands), hang it on the door as you recite this incantation:

Quiet and peace; disturbances cease.
Grant sleep and rest, so I can be at my best.

For pocket magic, bless your room key similarly, but change the incantation to reflect your goals. For example,

> *Don't bother me; stay away.*
> *I want privacy today.*

Since you'll be carrying your key with you, it will provide a magical buffer zone of privacy that will help you avoid any undesired company.

RED TAPE REMOVAL:

Are your travel plans buried under a mound of red tape, or do they seem to be running into a proverbial brick wall of problems? Try this spell to untangle things. Take seven strands of red thread or string. Bundle them up into your strong hand and focus on the difficulties you're experiencing. Let your tension drain into the string.

Now, open your hand and draw out one piece of string at a time, repeating this incantation with each thread: *"Troubles be gone, difficulties released. As I untangle this string, all problems shall cease."* Put the thread in a fireproof container and burn it, to likewise burn away the problems.

Carry the ashes in a sachet or other container. Then whenever the red tape starts getting tangled again, release a pinch of the ash to a wind blowing away from you. This will carry away the difficulties.

SUNSHINE ON MY SHOULDERS:

No one wants a vacation filled with rain. I remember one holiday in Oregon when I bought a T-shirt that read, "Oregonians don't tan, they rust!" That was understating how wet the vacation was.

To protect yourself from bad weather, carry a clove of garlic wrapped in a yellow or golden cloth (the color of sunlight). Empower this charm by adapting a children's rhyme,

Rain, rain stay away,
come again some other day;
clear the skies, I want to play!

Touch the charm and recite the incantation anytime the clouds threaten to rain on your parade.

POWER SHOPPING:

There is nothing more satisfying than finding wonderful souvenirs and trinkets at good prices. This amulet is for the budget-minded traveler who wants to be sure of purchasing quality products or services without overstretching their pocketbook. To make it requires two found pennies, a piece of malachite (for good deals), and a green cloth (the color of money). Prepare the amulet during a full moon, to likewise keep your pocket full.

Wrap the coins and the malachite in the green cloth, then pinch the coins between the thumb and index finger of your strong hand, saying,

A penny saved, a penny pinched;
saving money is a cinch.
On goods I find, the price shall fit
my pocketbook and wallet.

Carry this with you anytime you plan to go bargain hunting. After about three months, you should toss the pennies into a wishing well or fountain and refresh the charm with new pennies. The money collected at such places usually goes to charity, so your good fortune will bless others.

Alternative Components:

Anything you usually pack when traveling can become a component for powerful magic. Use the small bottles of shampoo for cleansing away negativity, use travel irons to smooth out difficulties, place an aromatic sachet filled with uplifting herbs in your travel bag, and anoint any tickets with a protective oil like myrrh or patchouli.

Once you arrive at your destination, observe everything in your hotel or motel room with a similarly creative eye. For example, use the ice bucket to cool an overheated temper and the shower cap as a component in a spell to keep bad weather at bay. In terms of timing, Wednesdays offer extra ingenuity.

Misdirected, Lost, and Found

This section covers those moments when the way you planned to travel isn't possible, or is temporarily blocked (for whatever reason). Second, it helps you find your way when you take a wrong turn at Albuquerque. Last, but certainly not least, it helps you locate lost wallets and other personal items that tend to stray at the worst possible moments, like when you have to pay a restaurant bill!

For divine blessing, consider the Greek goddess Gaia, who knows about everything that goes on around the earth and also presides over divination. So, she'll likely know *where* you need to go or *look* and *what,* if anything, you'll find when you get there! Alternatively, look to the Roman goddess Ops, a goddess of "opportunity" and luck.

TAKE THE LONG WAY HOME:

Suddenly you find your off-ramp is closed, your commuter flight canceled, or your bus route changed. Now what? With the Goddess's magic in your pocket, all is not lost. Make this charm and keep it handy for just such occasions.

Find any sort of dry seeds (Ops also presides over sowing) and put them in a sealable container. Take it in hand during a waxing moon to improve your luck, and bless it, saying,

> *Ops, bring your magic to me;*
> *help me find an opportunity*
> *to reach my destination with little fuss,*
> *be it by air, train, car, or bus.*

When you begin experiencing troubles, toss a few seeds to the birds, who will then carry your wishes on their wings, and then start exploring your "op-tions." Refill the container as needed.

IT DOESN'T LOOK LIKE KANSAS:

You're driving along, watching for landmarks, and you realize that nothing matches the directions you were given. You're lost, and, if you have luck like mine, there isn't a gas station or tourist stop in sight. Using the precept of "forewarned is forearmed," make this amulet in advance of any road trip to help avoid such problems, or to clear them up when they happen.

As the focus for this spell, I suggest using a Triple-A card, gas card, insurance card, or something similar that's likely to be in the car at all times. Take this token into the sunlight for clear thinking and say,

> *Token when touched, help me see the way;*
> *be empowered by the light of day.*
> *What once was lost, will soon be found,*
> *and I will be homeward bound.*

Whenever you feel lost, touch the token and repeat the incantation. If you are not going home, simply substitute your destination for the word *homeward*.

MAGICAL MAP MAGNIFIER:

This is a neat item to keep with you on the road to help with navigation, no matter what the circumstances. Find a small, hand-held magnifying glass. Charge it for five hours (the number of awareness) in both moonlight and sunlight. This enhances both the intuitive and the logical nature. Afterward, hold it in your hands, saying,

> *By night and by day,*
> *Gaia guide my way.*
> *Through this glass fine,*
> *let only accuracy shine!*

Use this to look over directions and maps anytime you're not certain of the right route to take.

TRAFFIC TALISMAN:

Why *do* we call it "rush hour" when no one gets anywhere? The traffic talisman is specifically designed to speed things along, or at the very least to keep them from halting altogether. It also acts to ward off accidents, which so often occur on crowded roadways.

On a Saturday, preferably when the moon is in Virgo for sound reasoning, take a jade stone (which protects against accidents that can be averted by attentiveness). Bind it to a morning glory (for patience). Drop a small amount of WD–40 on these two, to symbolically loosen things up. Wrap this with cloth and put it in your glove compartment. Whenever you reach an impasse, take the talisman out and put it on the dashboard, saying,

> Jade to keep safe along the way;
> morning glory to keep irritation at bay;
> oil to quicken, oil unbinds
> this traffic within which I am confined.

Continue chanting until the situation resolves itself. Tune up this talisman annually by adding a few more drops of oil. Note that if you carry this with you it can also work for busses and backed-up airlines.

WHERE, OH WHERE?

You're halfway home and realize something's missing. A purse, a pin, a tie, a coat . . . whatever the item, its loss can really spoil your whole day. This amulet is designed to help you reclaim those items that fall by the wayside, and to reduce future losses.

Start with a small magnet, a long piece of string, and a paper on which the name of the object is written. Wrap the magnet first with the paper, then with the string. Leave enough string unwrapped so that you can comfortably place the bundle across a table from you and hold the string in your hand. Focus your entire attention on the object, what it looks like, and the last place you remember seeing it. Slowly gather in the string as you whisper, *"Return to me."*

When the bundle reaches your hand, wrap it with the remaining string and carry it while you search. Once the item is recovered or replaced, burn the string and paper, with a prayer of thanks, and keep the magnet so that your other treasured possessions will always be attracted to you.

Alternative Components:

A map makes a perfect component in pocket magic for directional guidance, as does a compass. In the car, put a piece of jet on your dashboard to keep you safe against the dangers of the road. By boat, a moonstone keeps you true to course. Carry comfrey in your wallet for overall travel protection.

For possible timing, look to a full moon (especially one that occurs on a Monday) to improve your gut instincts and insight. The month of November enhances psychic awareness, and a moon in Libra aids discernment.

Auto-magics

For most of us, cars are nearly indispensable. Long gone are the days when a horse or two good feet provided all the transportation someone needed. Now we've grown accustomed to the welcome sight of a car waiting in the driveway to take us where we want to go, especially when it's raining! So, this section is dedicated to the one member of the family who listens unjudgmentally to our swearing at other drivers, and who stands at the ready to serve our commuting whims: our car.

To bless and energize your efforts, call on Epona, the Celtic horse goddess. Since horses were humankind's first mode of transportation, she seems a good choice to keep our "horse power" healthy and safe. To get Epona's attention, scatter corn kernels as an offering or leave out a cup of wine for her.

PARKING MAGIC:
Since I live in a city, I know all too well the evils of trying to park downtown. Either you can't find a space, or the lots are too expensive. There are two techniques that I advocate to overcome this problem.

The first is to take a handful of quarters, charge them in the light of a full moon for luck, and keep them in your car. The next time you need a parking spot, take one of the quarters in your hand and hold it up toward the sky. This is your offering to "De-meter," the goddess of good parking spots. Once you find a parking spot, feed "De-meter" her quarter. If you've found a free location, give this quarter to someone else's meter that's about to run out so the goddess gets her due, and you bless another's day!

Alternatively, several people I know use this invocation to find good parking: *"Great Sqat, I need a Spot!"* Chant this until a space opens up.

SPEED TRAP TALISMAN:
This spell is not intended to encourage anyone to break the law. Really, the best speed trap "magic" is using common sense. None-theless, there are some intentional speed traps, just waiting to ensnare the inattentive traveler. To avoid these problem spots, bless your radar detector, using a incantation like this one:

Show me where traps hide,
show me where traps wait.
Epona, stand by my side,
traffic tickets, abate.

Alternatively, you may want to dab your steering wheel with aromatics that help you stay alert, like lilac or rosemary. Recite the same incantation while you dab.

MECHANICAL FETISH:

I am among the mechanically challenged. So, I wanted to come up with a useful, portable charm that could help me in times of need. For my car I chose a fully functional tool kit, complete with extra fuses, bulbs, duct tape, and disposable damp cloths. The cloths are the focal point of the charm, but because they get stored with the rest of the tools, the magical energy saturates everything!

Put the cloths (baby wipes are one possibility) in a small, air-tight container. Put in a pinch of sage (for wisdom), a celery leaf or bit of caraway (for mental acuity), a mint leaf (for fresh ideas and to turn negativity), and some black tea (for the courage to at least *try*). Place this container in sunlight for one hour (the number of self-mastery). During the last minute of that hour, use this incantation:

> *Let me find my skill,*
> *let my eyes be keen;*
> *whatever the problems are,*
> *let them be seen!*

Put the container in your tool kit. Recite the incantation again each time you go to do a "quick fix." Let your higher senses guide you.

As an aside, these wipes come in handy anytime that you feel you need improved perspective on a situation.

THIEF, BEWARE!:

When I lived in South Boston, kids used to move my car every night as a joke (yes, they literally picked it up and moved it!). With growing numbers of people living in urban, and sometimes unsafe, environments, a little bit of magic certainly won't hurt to protect your car.

For this amulet you will need a Club or other anti-theft device. Alternatively, if these are too costly, use a piece of silver wire (or something silver-toned, like aluminum foil) bent to look like a pair of horns (to turn away bad intentions) and a small turquoise, which protects both the car and its owner in dangerous neighborhoods. If using wire, entwine the turquoise with it; if using aluminum, wrap the foil around it.

If possible, work during a waning moon, so that any undesired interest in your vehicle will also wane. Strongly visualize the token being filled with white-light energy as you say,

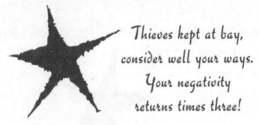

Thieves kept at bay,
consider well your ways.
Your negativity
returns times three!

If you are using an anti-theft device, make sure it's properly activated after you park your vehicle. Otherwise, keep this the token under a seat or in the glove compartment.

CAR BLESSING:

Take a protective aromatic with you to your car before driving, like garlic oil, onion juice, or dill pickle juice. Trace an invoking pentagram on the car's hood with the index finger of your strong hand (starting at the upper left and ending at the upper right of the star), while saying,

Epona, hear my prayer and bless
the North and South, East and West.
Whether I travel near or far,
keep me safe within this car.

Repeat this as often as desired. If no aromatics are available, use saliva, which has long been regarded as containing personal power.

Alternative Components:

Use anything that you take with you in the car regularly: traveling mugs for the water element (for "fluid" travel); a change holder for prosperity; sunglasses for keen insight; windshield fluid empowered to protect you from harsh elements; and child's car seats blessed for safety.

In terms of timing, most auto-magic moves well with a waxing to full moon for manifestation. Working on a Tuesday accents the conscious mind. Charms created in the month of August improve the harmony between you and your vehicle, and casting spells when the moon is in Sagittarius emphasizes wise mastery over this bit of technology.

Vehicle Venue

Thanks to the wonders of technology, our world offers numerous transportation alternatives. We can drive, take a train, go by bus, or fly in a plane or helicopter. Someday these options may even include spaceships! Consequently, our magic has to grow and change to meet the demands of a rapidly transforming, warp-speed culture. This section shares with you some practical ideas for pocket magic that affects vehicles other than your car.

The Goddess for vehicle magic is Inari, the Japanese fox goddess (sometimes a god), who presides over smithcraft (ironwork) and shape shifting, both of which are essential to the proper creation and maintenance of our modern vehicles.

BIKE AND MOTORCYCLE AMULETS:

Both bikes and motorcycles are terrific for sightseeing and low (or no) gas consumption, but they also expose the rider to dangers that a car does not. Since wearing a helmet in both instances has become the law in many states, I suggest using your helmet as the foundation for a practical amulet. Additionally, you will need a piece of masking tape on which you write the word *safety* or *protect*, as follows:

S	P
SA	PR
SAF	PRO
SAFE	PROT
SAFET	PROTE
SAFETY	PROTECT

This is a reversal of the format of the ancient charm Abracadabra, building positive energy. As you write, invoke Inari's blessing, saying,

Protection and shielding,
bound in this tape,
by Inari's power,
I shall always be safe.

Adhere the tape to the inside of the helmet. Repeat the invocation each time you put on the helmet.

AIRPLANE AMULET:

Since we don't have wings or feathers, some people are very queasy and nervous in airplanes. Even those of us who enjoy flying can feel safer when we carry a little bit of the Goddess with us. For this amulet you will need a small moonstone (which promotes protection and composure), a feather (which represents flight), and something to bind the two together. Take these in your hand, saying,

Inari, answer this behest;
security is my request.
When I travel 'cross the skies
keep me safe where'er I fly.

Bind the feather to the stone and keep it with you whenever you travel by airplane. Once a year make a new amulet, returning the old feather and stone to the earth with thankfulness.

TRAIN, BUS, AND SUBWAY TALISMAN:

Modes of public transportation have unique dangers, not the least of which are theft and assault. So, make yourself a practical talisman, using pepper spray as the base. Pepper is a protective, banishing herb because of its caustic quality.

Put the container in sunlight for seven hours to chase away shadows and negativity, and in moonlight for seven hours to improve your awareness. Then take it in both of your hands, visualizing bright, pure light filling it as you say,

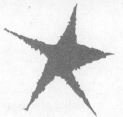

> *Protection, security, be with me;*
> *with this token, I claim safety.*

Attach this to your key chain so that it's always with you.

Alternative Components:

Magic components are vehicle-specific. On a bicycle or motorcycle, use side packs as a component to "hold" various types of energy, a horn for "making way," and a rear-view mirror you've blessed for keen vision. On a boat, use empowered motion-sickness pills for well-being.

In terms of timing, working on Thursday helps plans run smoothly, and the month of January improves foresight. Casting your spells when the moon is in Aquarius aids in personal enjoyment, and a waning moon emphasizes decreased difficulties.

Happiness Harbingers

Being able to predict the future by observing nature's signs is one of the oldest forms of divination. Since your eyes go with you on the road, put them to good use in mystically "seeing" what to expect from your trip.

For help with prophetic efforts, turn to Siduri, the Sumerian oracular goddess who also gives good advice. Pouring out a little ale will attract her attention. Alternatively, if you work on a Sunday, Tuesday, Thursday, or Saturday, call on Pingala, a Hindu divination goddess.

WHAT'S YOUR SIGN?
Think about your day for a moment. Can you think of something that you'd like more insight on? Concentrate on this question for about five minutes. Then, count to twelve slowly. The first traffic sign you see after the count represents your answer. Some sample interpretations include the following:

Stop: Problems ahead; consider an alternative route.

Bump: You're facing an obstacle that can be avoided or overcome.

Speed Limit: Slow down a little; you're missing something.

Curve: Change is on the horizon, so be aware.

No Shoulder: Some type of danger requires your full attention.

T Intersection: You are deciding between two equally appealing options. Choose carefully the path by which you walk.

Merge: You need to mingle more and integrate yourself without disrupting the flow that exists.

Traffic Circle: There is a repetitive cycle in your life; break the pattern if you desire change.

On-Ramp: A new opening presents itself.

A LICENSE FOR LIFE:

Following the same initial procedure as before, keep your question in mind, then make a mental note of the first license plate you see after counting to twelve. The numbers, letters, or both, can help you answer your question. Try adding together the numbers on the license plate for a numerical answer (see "Do It by the Numbers," in chapter 2).

If this number seems to hold no particular meaning, look at the letters. Do they spell a word? Are they the initials of someone you know who might be important to the question? Some letters, like I and O, have alternative meanings. I equals the self, and could mean that you are the key player in your question. O, like a circle, can represent protection or cycles.

COIN COLLECTOR CONGA:

For this bit of fortune-telling, you will need a coin cup and two coins of each denomination (two quarters, two dimes, two nickels, two pennies). Hold the cup in your hand and shake it as you would a dice cup, while thinking of your question. Close your eyes for a moment and say,

Siduri, guide my hand;
let your message before me land.

Tip the cup so it's at a diagonal, and shake it again until one coin pops out. This indicates your answer. Potential interpretations include the following:

Penny: Something's at stake here. This is the figurative "penny ante"; you have to invest something, but the risk to you is minimal.

Nickel: Watch your money. Make sure a person or a situation isn't nickel-and-diming you to death.

Dime: While we might lament that a phone call doesn't cost ten cents anymore, those days are gone. Likewise, you need to leave something from the past *in* the past.

Quarter: You need to communicate effectively or open the lines of discourse with someone.

The interpretive value of the coins can be increased by looking at the numerical value of the minting year. Alternatively, add coins from other countries and assign a significance to each for more variety.

Helpful Hint: keep the quarters and bless them for household magic (see "Quarter Quarters," in chapter 2) or "Parking Magic" (this chapter).

TREASURE HUNT:

Among some Native American tribes, finding objects (specifically natural ones) in unusual locations is considered to be a message from the Universe about a person's fate. So while you're traveling, watch to see if you find anything odd, unique, or distinctly out of place. The possible list of interpretive values is vast, considering how many things might fit into this category. So, here are just a few potential interpretations for your consideration:

Money: A good sign; improvements are coming, especially financial ones. Keep this and use it as a charm for abundance.

A black feather: Watch your health; don't exert yourself. Use this in a medicine bag for well-being.

Jewelry: There is a forthcoming social occasion that's formal. Bless and empower this for appeal.

A hat: Think about your choices before making a decision.

A ball: Take your turn "at bat" in a situation at hand. Throw it to a child with a wish for child-like joy.

A book: If you're thinking about learning something new, a book is a very good sign. Keep it around for when you have simple questions. Open it and read the first sentence you see for an answer.

A pin: If the point faces away from you, travel is on the horizon. Keep it for pocket magic centered on piercing charades and getting to the point.

A nail: A good omen; carry this for luck.

A candy wrapper: Read the print on this to see if it has an obvious meaning. For instance, "Almond Joy" can symbolize happiness. If so, use it as a component in a spell for joy.

When you find something, be it on this list or not, let your intuition and the Goddess's magic guide you in understanding the meaning. Try invoking her assistance by holding the item you've found and saying,

*Pingala, help me understand
your message, held within my hand.*

Keep repeating this phrase until you experience the lightbulb going on overhead, accompanied by that "Ah ha!" feeling.

BIRDS OF A FEATHER:

You know the old saying "a little bird told me"? Watch the birds to know what's going to happen while you're out and about! Birds flying on your right side, or toward the right, mean that a good day is ahead. Conversely, birds flying to the left portend difficulties. Mixed directions reveal that your day will have ups and downs that you can overcome through planning.

Blackbirds and bluebirds represent happiness. Crows are a bad sign. A duck indicates a new or refreshed love interest, eagles and hawks predict success, and a red bird means you will soon have a wish fulfilled.

If you're fortunate enough to have a bird drop a feather near you, pick this up and use it in your pocket magic!

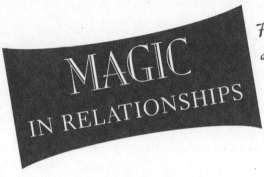

MAGIC IN RELATIONSHIPS

Familiarity breeds attempt.

—GOODMAN ACE

Whatever the era or culture, wherever you find incurable romantics, hopeful lovers, or Mr. or Ms. "afraid of commitment," you will also find the Goddess trying to help things along. Sure, the dating scene has changed a lot over the years. There are no knights in shining armor (other than those who arrive in a BMW), and the idea of "happily ever after" seems almost a work of fiction. Even so, love hasn't gone out of style. Everyone still needs to feel attractive to others, we still yearn for companionship, and the Goddess's magic is still around to help.

Wish that a passing acquaintance would make a real pass? Like to get that guy or gal across the room to look at you with more adoration than they do a cold beer on a hot day? Want to flirt with more than ideas? Then do just that! Hug the Goddess to your heart and let her energize your love affairs.

Gypsy Guidance

As a child, I remember tossing apple peels to divine an initial of the name of the person whom I would eventually marry. As a teenager, we played spin the bottle instead, hoping to jump-start a little interest. Then, as an adult, the dating game comes along—will it be number one, number two, or whoever's in the shoebox-sized apartment? Wouldn't it be nice if we just *knew* if someone would be a good or bad companion? A little magic can help!

This section is dedicated to spells that help us metaphysically discern the who, where, and when of relationships. Additionally, each spell has at least one portable component that will attract the right people to you at the right time.

Joe?
John?
Jim?

In matters of the heart, call on the Nordic goddess Freyja, who rules over love, wisdom, foresight, and a little luck (which never hurts). Freyja can be represented with feathers, cat images, a hawk, or heady perfumes.

SWEET DREAMS, BABY:

One of the most ancient ways of foretelling the future was through divinely inspired dreams. In this case you will be combining magical herbs known for producing prophetic visions with a prayer to the Goddess for assistance.

Make a small sachet filled with marigold and rose petals. Take this outside beneath a full moon. Look up, saying,

> *Freyja, hear my wish for dreams*
> *whilst I stand in your moon's beams.*
> *Bend down your ear from high above;*
> *help me find my one true love.*

Put the sachet under your pillow at night when you want to dream of potential lovers. During the day, carry it with you so that the Goddess can open the way for your magic to start manifesting.

MIRROR, MIRROR ON THE WALL:

Die-hard romantics say that for every soul there is a companion who reflects our heart's desires as closely as a mirror reflects our image. Taking this idea a little further, find a handheld mirror, preferably one that you can carry with you. During a waxing to full moon, draw a clockwise spiral around the mirror's glass with sandalwood oil, moving from the outside edge inward.

As you trace the circle, repeat this incantation until you reach the center:

Within this mirror my wish is sealed;
my lover's face, be revealed.

Observe the surface of the mirror for any symbols or images. Anything that materializes will have something to do with a future love. For example, if you see red-colored clouds, your mate might have red hair or favor the color red. If you see a building, that may be where they live, or where you will meet.

Carry the mirror with you to keep the vibrations of your wish activated.

APPLE PEELS AND SEEDS:

Several spells from the Victorian era recommend the use of apple peels and seeds for learning about your future love(s). The apple peel is tossed over the right shoulder while thinking about your desire to find a mate. If it takes the shape of a number, this indicates how many days, weeks, months, or years it will be before that special someone comes along. If it takes the shape of a letter, that initial will be part of the person's name. When you're done, dry the apple peel and use it in incense or as part of a portable charm to attract loving energies to you.

Eat the apple to internalize a little extra self-love, which will improve your outlook, and save the seeds. Toss these on a fire source, saying,

> Apple seeds that pop and fly,
> show me where my true love lies.
> Freyja, hearken to my request:
> are they north or south, east or west!

The direction in which the majority of the seeds fly indicates the region in which you will meet this person. The number of seeds reveals how long it will be in days, weeks, months, or years.

These seeds can now go into your love charm to heat things up.

CRYSTAL CLEAR:
Find a pink quartz (the color of affection) that fits easily in the palm of your hand. Think about your desire to find a significant other. Close your eyes for a moment, saying,

Crystal spirit, who shall be
my true love? Bring them to me!
Wisps of light, tell me when
my romance will begin.
And where, o' where does my love lie?
Bring the truth before my eyes.

Open your eyes and look at the surface of the stone as sunlight (or candlelight, if available) dances off of it. Don't look at anything specific—just watch for clouds or images to form. These can take the form of letters, pictures, or symbols that will answer your inquiry. It's up to you to discern exactly what the images mean.

Afterward, carry the stone with you to help attract the right people to you.

Alternative Components:

Any portable divination tools like runes, casting stones, tea leaves, or a small tarot deck will help you get an overview of the prevalent energies in any circumstance. Eat eggs and grapes or drink dandelion wine to heighten your divinatory ability. Carry tin for luck and improved foresight, or an obsidian to provide you with well-founded instincts.

Divinatory efforts can be accentuated if timed for a full moon, a Monday, or when the moon is in Cancer, all of which accent the lunar nature. The month of September energizes mystical understanding.

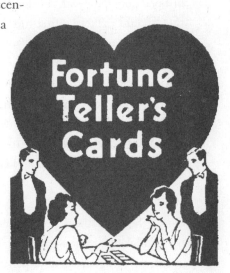

Charming Charms

Attracting the interest of another and holding onto that person has become a very tricky business these days. Gender-specific roles have been turned inside-out over a very short time, leaving most of us dazed and confused. Men don't know if they should pull out chairs or open doors, for fear of offending someone. Women aren't sure if they should make the first move. Parents haven't got a clue about what advice to give kids going on their first date!

While the old courting rituals have become passé, the Goddess can still help with the awkwardness of trying to attract an admirer's attention, and keeping that attention once you've got it. Venus, the Roman Goddess of attractiveness, love, and pleasure, is a good choice here. By improving self-esteem, Venus can help any wallflower learn to dance. Fred and Ginger, move over!

LOVE IS IN THE AIR:
One of the subtlest and easiest ways of attracting a mate is through the use of alluring aromas. Just as surely as fresh-baked bread grabs our attention, the right cologne or perfume can arouse "hunger" in another.

For this charm, find a sampler size of your favorite scent and a pink candle with a heart carved into it. Light the candle in a window where it will receive moonlight (preferably that of a full moon). Put the scent container in front of the candle, saying,

*Venus, grant me the love that I lack;
through this scent, my mate attract!*

Let the candle burn out naturally, then carry the scent with you, spraying on a little whenever you're in a social setting. You can energize the magic further by repeating the invocation when you don the perfume.

By the way, if you have a good, airtight container, you can also make your own love-attracting oils by adding essential oil to an almond oil base a few drops at a time until you like the scent. Engaging aromatics include cinnamon, ginger, jasmine, lemon, orange, vanilla, and rose.

LOOKING FOR LOVE (IN ALL THE WRONG PLACES):

Long-term companions are rarely found at singles bars. So, the question becomes, Where does one look for love? At museums, concerts, bowling alleys? All possibilities, but even when you can meet people with common interests, it's still hard to single out specific prospects. That's where this amulet can help.

Find a pair of rose-tinted sunglasses and wash them in lavender soap for heightened spiritual awareness (this helps you recognize people who have the right "vibes"). As you wash them, say,

For those who make passes, remove the rose-colored glasses;
their true nature discerned, from lessons I've learned.
When out on a date, I'll perceive a good mate.
When out on my own, scoundrels leave me alone.
No matter the hour, Venus, release your power!

Wear these when going out to meet people, but take them off just before scanning any room so that the "rose-colored glasses" literally get removed.

RING MY BELL:

You give someone your phone number, but will they *ever* call? If you're feeling a little impatient, try this talisman. On a piece of paper, write the name of the person you want to call you. Do this during a waxing moon to encourage growing communication. Adhere a piece of mica (which improves discourse) to the paper, reciting this incantation seven times (for fulfillment):

> *Venus, answer my plea;*
> *have _____ call or come to me.*
> *When, at last, we talk and share*
> *let your magic fill the air.*

Fill in the blank with the name of the person. Leave this talisman under your telephone (or modem) when you're home to get a call. Otherwise, carry it with you to increase the likelihood of bumping into the person and having a terrific time when you do.

WISHES ON THE WINDS:

This is a very useful spell because you can use it to send *any* wish out to the Universe. Simply change the base component to one suited to your desire. You will need about a cup of rose petals and lavender. Take these outside on any day when southerly winds are blowing (for passion). Slowly release half of this mixture while turning clockwise and saying,

> *South and West, North and East,*
> *Let this magic never cease*
> *until it finds my soul's mate,*
> *the one with whom I'll share my fate.*

Keep the remainder with you, releasing a pinch anytime you're near running water, or when you feel a warm breeze. The water conveys your wish out from you, while the warm breeze inspires warm feelings.

CURING DATE DREAD:

Okay, you finally meet someone you want to ask out on a date, but your backbone can't be found anywhere. What do you do? Go back to the Goddess's pocket and pull out some poise, starting with this charm.

Start by buying an aerosol breath freshener, preferably a spearmint-flavored one (spearmint is an herb of love and attraction). Take this in your hand, visualizing yourself conversing with the person, including asking them out. Add an incantation like the following:

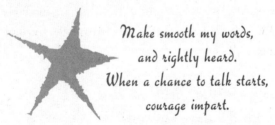

Make smooth my words,
and rightly heard.
When a chance to talk starts,
courage impart.

The next time you get a chance to approach this person, spray a little of the breath freshener in your mouth and go for it! You can also use this incantation any other time you need bolder speech.

THE FAIRY GODMOTHER:

Ever wish that you had a fairy godmother to open all the right doors? This little fetish is designed to draw a little fairy glamour into your life. First, on the first night of a full moon leave a small bit of cream and a sweet cake out on a window sill. This acts as an offering to the fairy folk and invites their presence to help with the creation of the fetish.

On the second night of the full moon, you will need something to act as a wand. This can be a pen, a children's toy wand (the ones with stars suspended inside), or even a toothpick with a gold star attached. Whatever your choice, it should be portable. Take the chosen object outside, and point it toward the moon, saying,

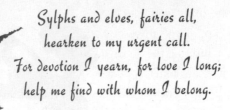

Sylphs and elves, fairies all,
hearken to my urgent call.
For devotion I yearn, for love I long;
help me find with whom I belong.

Carry the wand with you when you're in social situations. If you can leave out another small gift for the fairy folk each time you use the wand, all the better.

Alternative Components:

Empower your clothing to make it more alluring. Wear charged crystal jewelry (amber, cat's eye, and jasper are good choices for sex appeal). Sprinkle your shoes with energized fairy dust (glitter) so that you shine all the more when in the public eye.

For timing, work during a waxing to full moon to bring things to fruition. Wednesdays accent whimsy, the month of August improves harmony between people, and a moon in Aquarius cultivates enjoyment. Other good days for this spell are the traditional festival days for Venus, which included April 28, May 23, June 19, and August 9. Her day is Friday, which is dedicated to all relationship issues, especially love.

Tying the Knot

Keeping relationships healthy takes a lot of work, patience, and a big dose of level-headedness. Even with all the right ingredients, relationships are rarely picture-perfect. So, to kindle a deeper level of devotion, to ignite oneness, and to keep things fiery, add a spark of the Goddess's magic.

This type of pocket magic is intended for two willing, knowing participants. For divine assistance, we turn to Lakshimi, the Indian goddess of love, beauty, good fortune, and success. Lakshimi is also portrayed as the wise, devoted companion of Vishnu. Her flowers are the lily and the lotus.

LOVE POTION #9:

Take two cups of apple juice and add three strawberries and three raspberries (representing both of you, your unity, and joy), two orange slices (for devotion), one lemon slice (for fidelity), a pinch of ginger (for energy), and a pinch of sugar (for sweet feelings). Warm this over a low flame, then chill it.

Share the potion with your significant other beneath starlight or by candlelight. As each of you hands the drink to the other, say,

By accepting this cup, you accept my love,
as it is freely given.

Stare deeply into each other's eyes as you drink, then let nature take its course.

Retain the remaining liquid in two equal-sized, airtight containers (one for each of you). Dab it behind your ears or on your pulse points anytime you think fondly of your partner to extend those warm feelings to them, no matter where they may be. Just make sure to throw away the juice when it starts to turn. You don't want your love to get similarly moldy!

UNITED DESTINY:

Ancient gypsy tradition says that if two people wish to link their destiny, they should drink from one glass, then break it so that the promise can never be undone. You can use this tradition to empower the previous spell, or use it in another magically inspired moment.

One good time to use this symbolism is after a fight, as part of the healing process. Rededicate yourselves to working together by sharing some passion fruit juice. Pour any excess juice into a separate container with some alcohol to preserve it (symbolically preserving the passion), then break the glass you drank from. Collect the shards (carefully) and put them into a glass jar. Each person should then take a turn whispering into the jar any residual resentments they have toward the other. Then close the jar tightly and bury it to put the past behind. Keep the excess juice, dabbing a little over your heart anytime you feel the negativity from that argument returning.

LOVE COMFORTER:

Start with any large blanket with a soft, cuddly texture. Get some iron-on patches from the supermarket or a sewing outlet. From these, cut several hearts, or any other form that you associate with positive, loving emotions. Retain the scraps.

Follow the directions given on the package for properly ironing these onto the blanket; the best time to do this is during a full moon. The iron provides warm feelings, while a full moon helps bring maturity to a relationship. As you iron, say an invocation like this one:

> *Lakshimi, see our hearts.*
> *Keep our love strong, yet gentle, warm, and welcoming.*
> *When we share this cover, inspire comfort and kindness*
> *and dreams of each other.*
> *So be it.*

You can cut out one or two more patches of this material from the scraps and iron them onto items you wear regularly (like underwear) to carry this special warmth with you.

ROMANCE REFRESHER:

Hope to put a little fire under relationships that have grown downright chilly? Let the Goddess help. Plan this magic for an evening when the two of you can be assured of privacy. Begin with a metaphysically inspired meal, consisting of foods for love and passion (such as fish, sweet potatoes, beets, and apple-almond pie). Eat the meal by candlelight, using deep red candles anointed with banana essence or olive oil (both improve sexual interest).

Next, the two of you should move into a more comfortable space, each bringing a magnet. Sit facing each other (you may wish to undress first), each of you extending a magnet toward your partner, and whisper the following incantation three times:

Love and trust, passion's a must.
Pleasure extend, our relationship mend;
to both body and heart, desire impart.

As you repeat the incantation, slowly move the magnets together so they touch. Now let nature take her course. Both partners can carry their magnets to keep the power of attraction with them. Whenever either of you wants an intimate moment, you have but to leave the magnet on the refrigerator as an inspirational cue.

KEEP THE HOME FIRES BURNING:

Every living space is changed by those who live in it. One good way to symbolically and magically keep love alive at home is through the use of self-contained candles (those that are either set in an enclosed container or come in glass). Find a good supply of these, and anoint each one with a mixture of clove- and rose-scented oils.

On the first night after a dark moon (when the first crescent can be seen) light the first candle, saying,

> *Lakshimi, this candle represents our love*
> *and the spirit of unity in our home.*
> *As it burns, keep devotion and adoration burning*
> *in our hearts.*

When it looks like this candle is about to burn out, immediately replace it with the next, repeating the invocation. Keep these burning at all times (if possible and safe) as a constant reminder of the Goddess's presence and blessings.

Retain the wax from the first candle. When it has cooled slightly, fashion yourself a small wax heart from it. Write the name of your partner in the wax and carry it with you as a charm to keep love vibrant.

Alternative Components:

Apply your partner's favorite cologne to keep them with you when traveling, or wear the scent they prefer on you to invite their attentions. Carrying beryl, lapis, or pink tourmaline, or burning rose, vanilla, or jasmine incense regularly keeps the vibrations of love in and around your life.

Consider enacting your spells on Valentine's Day, anniversaries, birthdays, and other special days associated with your relationship. Fridays, the month of June, and when the moon is in Pisces are all times that accentuate the vibrations of love, devotion, and romance.

Passion and Pleasure

Not all of us have the bedroom savvy we might like. Everybody experiences moments of awkwardness or of feeling downright silly. In this case, laughter is actually good medicine for what ails you. It releases a lot of tension. I also prescribe adding the Goddess's magic to make your romantic meetings all the more memorable.

Two lusty ladies hold potential for this type of magic. The first is Lilith, the Babylonian and Sumerian seductive goddess of erotic dreams and forbidden delights. The other is the ever-tantalizing Aphrodite, the Greek goddess of sexual love.

LOVE IN THE AFTERNOON:

During the day before a planned passionate encounter, both people should lunch lustily. This means packing a special meal specifically designed and empowered to promote desire. It could include deviled eggs, clam chowder, cardamom-seasoned rice, and blackberries. Gather your chosen edibles together and hold your hands over them, palms down, saying,

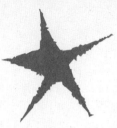

Lilith, Aphrodite,
inspire passion and delight.
Let what we eat this afternoon
enliven rapture tonight!

Portion out the meal equally, giving half to your partner in a brown bag complete with a bawdy note. If you can't do this, set half aside to symbolically keep the passionate energy waiting for their arrival.

MASSAGE IN MEANING!

Sometimes rushing into sexual situations dampens people's interest. When this happens, try using a magical massage oil to liven things back up. Make this by steeping catnip (for beauty), a slice of lemon (for friendly feelings), a pinch of marjoram (for enjoyment), and a vanilla bean (for passion) in one cup of warm almond oil during a full moon. Visualize the oil being filled with bright red light as you chant,

Rekindle desire,
relight the fire.
Through my heart and my hand,
let passion extend.

Allow this chant to increase in volume naturally until the entire room vibrates with power. Store the oil in a portable, airtight container to draw the energy of pleasure to you. Warm it up before applying it. As you gently trickle the oil on your partner, mentally recite the incantation again to release the magic.

ALL NIGHT LONG:

Have a big night coming up and want to still be interested in your partner come the wee hours of the morning? Make yourself a staying-power fetish. Gather together two capers, a dried radish, celery seed, a sprig of parsley, and a pinch of ginger. These herbs are for energy, lust, and sexual prowess.

Next, take an unlubricated condom and bundle the herbs inside it (for safe sex). Leave this in sunlight for three hours (for alertness), and in moonlight for three hours (for romance). Bless this fetish, saying,

Lady of love, great Aphrodite,
empower this fetish,
grant me energy and passion through the night!

Keep this token in your pocket or some other discreet location when you go for your rendezvous.

A TEASING TALISMAN:

This pocket magic is excellent for playful relationships. Buy a couple of large, soft feathers. These can often be found at Asian import shops or craft stores. When the moon is in Aquarius (to inspire adventure), take the feathers in your hand and begin wrapping the quill ends together using a bright red satin ribbon. Crisscross the ribbon around the quills, knotting it at each cross mark. As you make the knots, say,

Pleasure and fun,
I aim to please.
With enticement and passion,
these feathers will tease!

When you reach the bottom of the quills, tie off the ribbon securely. Make sure you have this with you when you and your partner retire. Tickle their aura and body gently with it to arouse desire. Keep it handy to inspire playfulness during lovemaking.

Alternative Components:

Simmering potpourri filled with energized herbs will warm things up. Quartz crystals around the bedroom will keep physical energy at an optimum. Eat sensual foods, like cream-covered strawberries, that you have blessed, then feed them to each other. Wear sexy undergarments scented with lusty aromatics.

Magic for passion benefits from nighttime casting, because of the night's romantic ambiance. However, portable items can be charged in sunlight to accent the fire element. A moon in Aquarius accents the spirit of adventure and pleasure.

Fertility Fever

Is your biological clock saying "tick"? Have you and your partner wanted a child, but been unsuccessful till now? The Goddess is an old hand at childbirth, being the mother to humankind (and of course, fertility can apply to more than just babies). The Goddess's special magic can provide just the right nudge to help nature (or physicians) along! Even when "natural" methods won't work, she assists with adoption procedures by opening the right doors.

For this, I recommend calling on Kwan Yin, the Chinese goddess of fertility, who is also called "she who brings children" or "she who hears the cries of the world." Her compassion is packaged together with impressive magical skills in a formidable lady who understands our heart's desires.

CONCEPTION CHARM:

Both partners should gather seven nuts and seven seeds along with a green cloth and a yellow string. Take these components outside when there's an easterly wind (for a new beginning). Bundle the seeds and nuts together in the green cloth (for growth). Tie the sachet with the yellow ribbon (for creative energy), knotting it seven times for completion. With each knot, say,

> Kwan Yin , see our hearts.
> To our bodies, your blessing impart.
> Fill these tokens with fertility;
> let our love manifest in pregnancy.

Carry these tokens in your pockets (near the groin) or close to your heart as often as possible. During lovemaking, keep one on each side of the bed. And don't overlook practical things, like getting lots of rest, eating well, and enjoying each other!

EGGS-ACTLY!

Eggs are an age-old symbol of fertility. In addition to eating them to internalize this energy, you can use them to make terrific charms. Start by hollowing out an egg (blow out the yoke and the white). Decorate the shell carefully, using symbols that represent conception to you.

On a small sheet of paper write your wish for a baby, and slide this into the shell. Leave the decorated egg in the light of a waxing to full moon for three nights, then move it to a makeshift cradle of soft fabric near your bed. Wait until the next waxing to full moon (or when the woman is fertile), and stand before the egg. Put your strong hands over it, allowing your bodies to be energized by your wishes and the growing moon. Make love with hopefulness!

ADOPTION AMULET:

The process of adoption can be long and heartrending. To make things move along more smoothly, create this amulet. It will protect you from undue obstacles and surround you with welcoming energy.

Begin with whatever paperwork you have on the adoption and three pink crystals (for gentle love). Put the crystals on top of the paperwork in a prominent spot at home. Nearby, keep a white candle burning to represent the Goddess's power. Bless this configuration, saying,

> *Lady, fulfill this wish:*
> *We open our hearts and our home to a young soul.*
> *Guide our efforts and hasten the way.*

Each partner should then carry one of the three crystals with them at all times to extend love and open doors for the right child to join them. Leave the remaining stone in place to energize the paperwork. Repeat your prayer whenever you replace the candle.

Alternative Components:

Use a statue of the pregnant Goddess as a fetish. Use coral and jade bound together for flowing fertility. Also use cradles and other items associated with preparing for the arrival of a child.

For timing, any day in the spring is good, when the earth shows signs of productivity. Mondays accent lunar energies (e.g., the feminine cycle), the month of April improves luck, and the moon in Virgo augments fruitfulness.

Preserving the Peace

When an ego gets overblown, when words are misunderstood, when folks get oversensitive, all manner of difficulties can result. No matter how well-meaning we might be, nobody's perfect. So when you open your mouth to change feet, take a moment to work a little magic, too.

Call on Nerthus, a Teutonic goddess, for aid in armistices. Traditionally, at her festivals no one could bear arms unless the weapon was peace-bonded (tied into its sheath), and any public arguments were severely reprimanded. She can help us sheath our harsh words and actions.

TACTFUL TONIC:

If you're going to swallow your words, they might as well be tasty. Begin with a cup of hot black tea (for calming). Add to this one-fourth teaspoon coconut flavoring (for restraint), a one-eighth-inch slice of ginger root (for positive energy), one teaspoon pineapple juice (for protection and harmony), and a shot of peach brandy (for warmth and wisdom). Stir the ingredients clockwise, saying,

When on my lips this liquid drops,
anger end; hostility stop.
Words be gentle, words be kind,
help me speak the truth that's on my mind.

Drink half the cup before talking over the problem. Keep the other half in a breakproof portable container. Dab a little on your throat chakra anytime you need to improve communications.

FORGIVENESS FEAST:

This is basically a mini-ritual. Each person involved in a dispute brings to a neutral location one dish to be shared (like at a potluck supper), one candle, and one white flower. The food should somehow represent the desire for peace (like mashed potatoes, because they're white and smooth). Situate the candles around the feast table, with the flowers in the middle, representing peace.

Before dinner, each person should blow out their individual candle to indicate their willingness to forgive and leave the past behind. As each person takes their turn, the others chant,

Anger released, hostility ceased,
we now create peace.

Each then takes up a flower to keep with them, extending a handshake or a hug to the other participants. The petals from the flowers should be dried for incense and charms that will engender harmony between people. Finally, dinner gets consumed to internalize the magic.

CEASE-FIRE!

It's hard to generate forgiveness when you can't be heard over the shouting. This talisman is designed to inspire cooler heads and warmer hearts. Take the image of a heart cut in two. By the light of a waning moon (to decrease hostility), apply some salve mixed with glue to the image. Put the two halves together, saying,

Calm the anger, calm the ire,
cool the raging inner fire.
Let forgiveness replace fury and fear
between me and the one that I hold dear.

Carry this token with you the next time you meet with the person to try to work things out. When the problem finally resolves itself, wrap the heart in a satin cloth and keep it somewhere safe to continue encouraging peaceful love.

EXIT STAGE LEFT:

Some arguments defy rectification to the point where a relationship dissolves. Most people would prefer that such breakups weren't dramatic and heart-wrenching. This amulet is meant to help on both counts. It protects the bearer from unnecessary heartache and opens the path for peaceful separations.

To create this amulet you will need a pair of scissors, a small doll (dollhouse size), and a length of string that can go around your waist two times. During a dark moon (the time of endings), tie the string around your waist once, and attach the small doll to the other end of the string. If possible, put something on the doll that belongs to the individual you're breaking up with, so it better represents his or her energy.

Put the doll across from you, and speak to it like you would speak to that person. Tell it your feelings honestly. When you feel completely done, take the scissors and cut the string away from your waist, saying,

I free you; I free myself
without malice or regrets.
Our lives have touched in peace;
now they part in peace.

Wrap the string around the doll and carry it with you to the fateful meeting. Afterward, you may wish to bury it to likewise bury any lingering negativity.

DON'T GET MAD, GET EVEN:

When Mr. or Ms. Right has proven to be totally wrong, unfaithful, or deceptive, there is a natural desire to get even. But old curses like *"May the fleas of a thousand camels inhabit your pubis"* seem out of place these days. So, instead, use this spell to get that person's karma working in your favor.

Take any picture you have available of the person's face, along with a small mirror. Glue the image face-down on the mirror's surface, saying,

> *Nerthus, my prayers heed.*
> *The harm _____ intended, return times three.*
> *Let him/her know firsthand what he's/she's done to me.*
> *Let my heart heal, and from sadness be freed.*

The nice part about this charm is that it returns only *intended* evil, not things that someone did unintentionally. Carry the charm with you until you feel the pain of that experience leave you. Then throw it away as unnecessary baggage from the past.

Alternative Components:

Use white candles, clothing, or other white items to indicate a truce. Lettuce salad with olives and creamy dressing will internalize tranquillity. Use any object that reminds you of the value of flexibility, like rubber bands.

In terms of timing, look to a waning moon to decrease anger and resentment. Casting spells as the sun set helps leave negativity behind you, while sunrise marks a fresh start. Working on a Tuesday will improve your sense of logic, while a Saturday will help manifest outcomes. The month of August cultivates a sense of unity, and the moon in Aries breaks down the barriers between people.

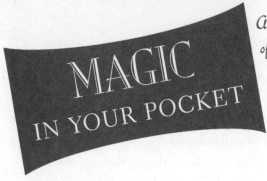

MAGIC IN YOUR POCKET

An empty pocket's the worst of crimes!
—CHARLES P. SHIRAS

Amulets, charms, talismans, and fetishes are the ultimate expressions of portable magic. By making and carrying these items we, like our ancestors, reclaim the Goddess's power and take it with us to where it's most needed. Some people have lucky coins or hats. Others refuse to go into a meeting without a specific mug, pen, or clipboard. Whatever the object, the intent is the same—to energize and enjoy our day more through fulfilling magic.

Harnessing Health

As the old saying goes, "If you have your health, you have everything." Feeling good makes life's other turbulence much easier to bear. Magic is also more successful when it's created by a healthy person who can devote 100 percent of their focus and energy to the matter at hand.

Invoke the assistance of Salus, the Roman goddess of health and welfare. Her festival day was January 1, perhaps with the idea of getting the year off on a good physical footing. The Greek equivalent is Hygeia (note the modern English word *hygiene*), daughter of the god of health and sister of Panacea, a goddess of life-promoting elixirs.

SEEING RED:
Because our blood is red, ancient people believed this color could scare away the mischievous spirits that caused sicknesses, especially colds. All that's required is wearing a red scarf regularly. If you live in a fluctuating climate, bless one dress scarf and one winter scarf for year-round protection. To do this, take the scarves in your hand during a waning moon (to banish the power of disease) and say,

> *Salus, let this cloth of red*
> *banish all sickness from my bed.*
> *This magic cleans where'er germs dwell;*
> *throughout the year, I will be well!*

Wear these regularly to keep sickness at bay.

TURNING OVER A NEW LEAF:

A wonderful bit of Victorian lore says that if you catch an autumn leaf as it falls from the tree (before it hits the earth) you will be free of colds all winter. Keep this leaf as a protective amulet and empower it, saying,

> *I'll get relief from all colds,*
> *because this leaf, my magic holds.*
> *Sniffles and sneezes cannot win;*
> *when I carry this leaf, the magic begins.*

Now, preserve the leaf by ironing it between two sheets of waxed paper (waxed side toward the leaf). The heat activates and energizes the magic. Carry it with you throughout the cold and flu season.

THE CRYSTAL CONNECTION:

The ancients carried all manner of crystals, believing that each stone had an indwelling spirit that could protect them from illness. Building on this idea, make yourself a healthy medicine bag by combining one piece each of amber, eye agate, turquoise, jade, and coral into a portable satchel. Each of these stones ensnares sickness, protects you from it, and encourages physical wholeness. Leave the pouch in the light of the sun (considered healthful) for three hours (the number of body, mind, and spirit).

Each time you feel yourself growing weary or feeling under the weather, put the pouch in your pocket, saying,

Amber traps the malady.
Agate keeps my spirit free.
Turquoise turns away calamity.
Jade from sickness keeps me free.
With the coral neatly bound, renewed health will soon
be found.

Continue carrying the medicine bundle until you feel totally recuperated.

HERBAL HARMONY:

The components in this talisman are proportioned to make enough healthful sachets so that you can put one each in the bedroom, the kitchen, and the car, and still have one to carry with you. This way you can surround yourself with the energy of wellness.

Gather four teaspoons each of rosemary, mint, fennel, and apple rind (dried and diced). You will also need one strand of saffron per sachet (for emotional health and increased energy). Cut out four 4-by-4-inch green pieces of cloth and four white ties (ribbon or thread). During a waxing moon (for improved health), place equal amounts of the herbs in each sachet, saying,

> One, for body; two, for soul;
> three, for mind; four, keep me whole.
> Hygeia, empower this simple spell;
> energize these talismans to keep me well.

Put three of the talismans in areas where you spend a lot of time, and carry the fourth with you always.

IN THE PINK:

Using this phrase as a foundation for healthful magic, when you feel a little under the weather, don any pink garment. Eat a breakfast that includes pink grapefruit juice that's energized with a simple prayer, like *"Let health abound; keep my body sound."* Drink the juice to internalize the energy.

For a portable amulet that supports this magic, take a handful of red beans and bless them as you did the juice. In Japan these are considered potent health protectors.

LAUGHTER IS THE BEST MEDICINE:

The ancient Romans really took this idea to heart by creating an entire holiday dedicated to laughter: Hilaria, on March 25. So, on or around this date, set aside a little time just for fun. Dig out the silliest picture you can find of yourself (perhaps one of those used as bribery material, or taken at unaware moments). Cut it down so you can carry it in your wallet, and then enchant it by saying,

When a smile cannot be found,
raillery, herein be bound.
Laughter be quick, laughter be kind,
laughter, bring relief to my weary mind.

Put the picture in your wallet and look at it anytime you start taking yourself or life too seriously.

ALL TIED UP:

A very popular type of amulet in Arabia consisted of knots, using the symbolism of capturing and holding energy. For this amulet, you'll need a bit of netting, such as cheesecloth that is used to strain out unwanted substances. Leave the cloth in sunlight for four hours to absorb healthy qualities. Then make four evenly spaced knots in the cloth, saying,

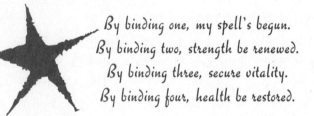

By binding one, my spell's begun.
By binding two, strength be renewed.
By binding three, secure vitality.
By binding four, health be restored.

Carry this with you. When you start feeling under the weather, untie one knot to release the magic. When you've used three of the four knots, refresh the amulet by leaving it in sunlight again, and retie the three knots while repeating the incantation.

Alternative Components

Dab on health-supporting aromatics like sandalwood, rose, and lotus. Wear green regularly, or wear another color you associate with well-being. Pray over your meals. Carry an ankh, the Egyptian emblem of life, or other personally significant magical symbols.

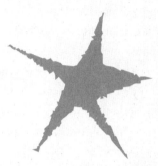

Create your talismans by a waning moon to decrease illness, or by a waxing moon so that health will grow. Working on Sunday accents solar, healthy energy. According to the Chinese calendar, the month of May improves vitality.

Jumping for Joy

Got a case of the "I don't care" blues? Feeling as if *nothing* you do makes any difference? If so, you've been bitten by the apathy bug, and you need a magical booster shot. Your physician for combating this case of indifference is the Goddess, and there's no waiting for an appointment!

Call on Bast, the Egyptian cat woman, to foster the enjoyment of life's every moment. Of all animals, cats truly know how to have fun and relax. Taking many attributes from her sacred animal, Bast represents pleasure, jokes, playfulness, kindness, and happiness.

AROMA THERAPY:

Remember the red scarf for health? It can do double duty now as a component to improve emotional health. Dab a little lavender oil on the scarf either when the moon is waxing (to cultivate joy) or during the day (so light banishes the "dark clouds"). As you work the aroma into the fabric, say,

> *Bast be gentle, Bast be kind,*
> *lift the burdens lying heavy on my mind.*

Renew joy, pleasure, and levity
so my spirit can fly free.

Wear this as often as possible until your mood improves. Change the aromas to suit other needs in your life: for instance, use pine for prosperity and sandalwood for psychic ability.

UP, UP, AND AWAY:
Get a bag of children's balloons. Take out all the blue ones. Put these together, hold your hands over them, palm down, and say,

Lift my heart, blues be kept at bay
when these balloons fly away.
Lift my spirits, higher still.
Bast, my magic wish fulfill.

Anytime you feel sadness or depression getting the best of you, blow up one of the balloons, repeat the incantation, then release the end so it flies away from you while deflating. In the interest of not harming animals that might eat the balloon, pick it up afterward and discard it properly. This also symbolically throws away the negative feelings.

IT'S BLOWIN' IN THE WIND:

Air is a powerful element for change, and it's something that's around you all the time—so it's a perfect vehicle for pocket magic. If you've been feeling melancholy, try to wait until the winds are blowing from the south (for cleansing) or from the west (for healing). Take a piece of blue cloth or ribbon and tie it *loosely* to a clothesline, bush, tree, or your mailbox, saying:

> *I leave here my sadness, and a heavy heart.*
> *When freed by the winds, melancholy depart!*

By the time the wind loosens the ribbon or cloth, you should find yourself feeling much better.

When you're out and about, always have a few fabric remnants or ribbons handy in your pocket magic kit. Ones of different colors can be used similarly, but applied for different needs. For example, use green ribbon for wishes relating to finances and change the invocation to something like *"When this ribbon freely flies, soon thereafter money arrives!"*

I'M TICKLED:

Combine a little creative visualization with a magically empowered feather, and you should soon find the blues lifting. Hang a large white feather in a window where it can receive energy from easterly winds (which symbolize new beginnings and hope) for three days. Afterward, take it in your hand and imagine it filled with white, cleansing light as you say,

Make me laugh, let joy be mine.
Within my aura, let your light shine!

Gently move the feather through your auric field from head to toe, and literally tickle yourself happy! Carry it with you so it's handy anytime you feel a little down.

CHARMED, I'M SURE:

To promote the vibration of happiness in and around your life, make this charm. Begin with a number of small amethyst crystals (for increasing your sense of peace, soothing raw nerves, and decreasing stress) and a container to house them in. Soak the stones in saltwater to clear their energies, then leave them in sunlight for a while (for warmth and comfort). Carry the container with you as part of your magic kit.

When you start feeling disheartened, take out one of the stones. Hold it in your hand, allowing all of your negative emotions to pour into the crystal. Give it your pain, your sadness . . . all the excess emotional baggage that you don't need cluttering your life. When you feel empty, throw the stone as far away from you as possible, saying,

Gone from me, all negativity.
Happiness to me; joy be free!

Accept the energy of happiness as it flows back to you. Do not look to see where the stone went; you don't need it anymore, and the earth takes care of her own.

Alternative Components:

Wear energized scents like apple blossom, lilac, and basil to encourage joy. Don your favorite colors or whimsical clothing to liberate your inner child. Along the same lines, toys and games can relieve stress and release the power of playfulness.

Work during daylight or on Sunday; the sun is a symbol of happiness and divine blessing. The month of April accents spring's upbeat energy, August promotes inner peace, and the moon in Aquarius emphasizes enjoyment.

Luck Lore

There is no such thing as too much luck. Good fortune is something we all hope for but don't always receive. These charms and amulets are designed to manifest serendipity in your life on a more regular basis.

For assistance in luck magic, turn to Gefun, the Nordic goddess of fortunate events, whose name means "the giver." Alternatively, consider the Morae of Greek tradition, three goddesses who ruled destiny. Specifically, Lachesis presided over the element of chance in every soul's life.

GET OFF ON THE RIGHT FOOT:

For whatever reason, people have always thought there was something special about the right side of the body. Your body is the one thing you can be sure of having whenever you need it. So, when bad luck seems to be following you around, each time you start walking always get off on the right foot, literally! To empower this action even more, keep a tiny piece of tin in your right shoe, and dust both shoes with lucky foot powder (baking soda, allspice, and nutmeg). Finally, dab a little pomegranate juice on the sides of your shoes as you say,

> *Hospitality and luck wherever I roam,*
> *then good fortune follows when I return home.*

Don't forget to make a wish when eating the pomegranate, for a little extra good fortune.

TURN IT AROUND:

A favorite Victorian way of changing bad luck was to symbolically turn it away by turning clothes backward or inside out (socks and underwear work well). You can try this yourself anytime you feel that luck is understocked in your life. To energize the magic further, perform this action by the light of the first star appearing in the night sky (and make a wish), or when the moon is waxing so luck grows. Add an incantation like this one:

> *Misfortune away, bad luck abate,*
> *by Gefun's power, a good change in my fate.*
> *When this fabric turns, so does destiny.*
> *Today I claim fortuity!*

If you don't feel comfortable turning around a piece of clothing, cross your fingers instead and change the incantation to

Bad luck, at the crossroads caught.
There it remains; good fortune I claim.

Keep your fingers crossed until you feel the negative energy has passed and improvements have started. If you can't cross your fingers for that long, cross any two portable objects and bind them together until the bad streak ends.

FOUND FORTUNES:

Finding things is considered very lucky, and therefore found objects make perfect tokens for portable luck magic. Bless found pennies and use them to scratch off your lottery tickets, and keep found keys to open luck's door. Pins can be empowered for times when you need to hold energy to yourself, and old nails can help with security magic. Whenever you find an object you feel you can use for this type of pocket magic, pick it up, saying,

See a _____ (name of object), pick it up!
All the day, I'll have good luck.
And when trouble might come my way,
this little _____ will bless my day.

Note that you can change the word *luck* to any word that better expresses your present needs or your magical intentions for that item.

BEAN BANISHING:

According to Eastern tradition, beans banish bad luck and sunflower seeds turn luck your way. So, gather a few dried beans and charge them in the light of a waning moon for reduced misfortune. Also gather some sunflower seeds, charged in sunlight to draw divine favor, and a portable container. Hold the seeds in the palm of your hands, saying,

> *When these seeds are planted in the ground,*
> *let luck abound and*
> *fortune turn around!*

When you need your luck to change, put one of each seed in good soil to grow. Refill the container as needed, but always leave one of each seed inside so that you never totally expend your good fortune.

JACK JUMPED OVER THE CANDLESTICK:

In Celtic tradition, crossing over a fire marks a transition—from sickness to health, from being single to marriage, and so forth. Using this symbolism, get a candle whose color represents luck to you. Dab it with a little orange juice (for good fortune). Light it and jump over it, saying,

> *Morae, you who weave the strands of fate*
> *change my luck, ill fortune abate!*

Keep some of the melted wax from this candle as an amulet for good luck. Carve an emblem into the wax to empower the magic further. One possibility is etching a sun, which represents hope.

STONE CERTAIN:

A favorite old way to encourage good luck was by carrying or wearing specific semiprecious or precious stones. One example that's still quite common is wearing one's birthstone. Since birthstones often prove rather costly, go to a science shop or New Age store and purchase a small tumbled obsidian, onyx, and jade instead. Put these in a pouch or other small container, repeating this incantation a personally lucky number of times:

> *Obsidian reflects misfortune away.*
> *Onyx keeps difficulties at bay.*
> *Jade, my good fortune increases.*
> *Blessed by Gefun, so luck never ceases!*

Carry this with you everywhere. If your luck gets worse, throw away either the obsidian or the onyx to move the bad luck away from you. Replace the stone later, reciting the incantation again to reestablish magical symmetry.

SERENDIPITY SACHET:

Besides stones, our ancestors often carried plants to invoke luck, since nature's supermarket was always open! To make this lucky sachet, you will need a four-by-four-inch piece of cloth cut from an old garment, so that the cloth already contains your personal energy. Fill the center of the cloth with a lucky number of allspice berries, hazelnuts, heather blossoms, and marigold petals. Leave this talisman in sunlight for a while (a personally lucky number of minutes), and empower it, saying,

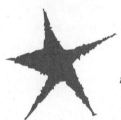

*As I place this in the sun,
so my magic is begun.
Herbs empowered with blessed light
cause all bad luck to take a hike!*

Carry this with you. When fortune takes a bad turn, sprinkle the herbs around you in a counterclockwise circle, repeating the incantation again to turn the negativity away. Refill the sachet later.

Alternative Components:

Wear aromatics like cinnamon and lotus, whose vibrations encourage better fortune. Put a piece of parsley, a bay leaf, or an ash leaf in your pocket or shoes. Eat poppy seed rolls or oranges to internalize lucky energy. And don't forget to think positively; gloomy thoughts attract bad luck.

Perform your spells in sunlight to invoke divine blessings. Work during a waning moon to banish misfortune, or a waxing moon so that luck will grow. The month of April increases fortune, and the moon in Pisces brings miracles.

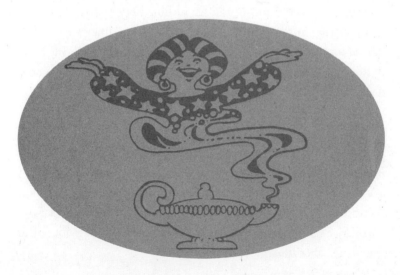

Love Baubles (Or Is that Boggles!)

Many people spend years chasing after love, perhaps the most elusive of emotions, and when they get it, they expend even more energy and effort making sure it's really theirs. The Goddess has watched this ongoing game of tag, and she knows the human heart well. She, and her magic, are the perfect helpmates to increase the amount of love in and around our lives. This includes self-love, which many people lack.

When you feel lost in the sea of humanity and really need a warm, caring anchor, call on Astarte, the Assyro-Babylonian goddess of love, marriage, sexuality, and oddly enough, war! She has a fighting spirit to aid your efforts to find love and to keep it safe once discovered.

CONDOM SENSE:

These days, practicing safe sex often goes hand in hand with searching for love. So why not modernize our magic by using condoms for a component, since both men and women can easily transport these? Leave the package of condoms in sunlight for three hours (to encourage sound thinking) and in moonlight for three hours (for romance). Then, energize them by saying,

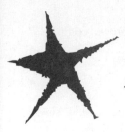

Astarte bless this little spell.
To my words, pray, listen well.
Love and passion, bring to my heart,
and with them wisdom, now impart.

Carry one or two of the condoms in your wallet or purse, or leave them in another easily accessible location. After you use them, get another from the package and put it in your purse or wallet so that desire is always balanced with discretion.

BREATH MINT MAGIC:

Want to make your conversation smoother and your words sweeter when approaching a companion? Use breath mints or mint gum as a component! Mint generates interest, arousal, and fresh energy.

Charge several packages in a southerly wind (for passion), so you have replacements ready when one is used up. If you like, add an incantation such as this one:

Let words be sweet, let words please,
let them encourage, invite, and tease!

Keep the candies with you as a talisman for improved communications.

CHAPSTICK CHARM:

To make yourself more "kissable" and desirable to your date or significant other, begin with Chapstick. Choose a flavor that is associated with love, like cherry. Hold the container in the hand that you normally extend when accepting an object from someone else. Symbolically, this extends an invitation to an intended individual. Repeat this incantation three times while thinking of one particular person:

When you look at me, you shall not miss
an opportunity to steal a kiss!

Put a little of the Chapstick on each time you're going to see this person, and repeat the incantation—then pucker up!

BELIEVE IT OR KNOT:

This charm begins with a piece of red thread (or use another color you associate with love). Bind it with five knots (one for each point of a pentagram). As you tie each knot, focus wholly on your intention to find a companion or improve your current relationship, saying,

With this thread of red I wind
magic for love, of a special kind.
Woven in each knot I make
feelings that cannot be faked.
When released, these will spark a fire
of trust, adoration, and desire.

Keep this thread with you and untie one knot whenever you feel you need more love. Take care, however, not to undo too many knots, too quickly. If love burns out of control, it will also burn itself out.

TAVERN TALISMAN:

In the dating game, we can't always be sure of the players. This token will keep away people who do not have your best interest at heart, while attracting those who might. For this talisman you'll need a small jar of avocado skin cream (for attractiveness); add to this a drop of rose-scented oil (for love) and a myrrh tear (for protection). If possible, add the myrrh and oil when the moon is in Gemini, to help bring diverse factors into agreement. Stir the cream clockwise, saying,

Let the beauty within shine without.
Astarte, erase my fears and doubts.
Let those who care little, quickly depart;
to those who care much, I extend my heart.

Keep this container with you. Rub a little on your hands (before shaking hands) or on your face (for physical comeliness) just before meeting someone new.

IMAGE-INATION:

One of the hardest things in relationships is being able to see ourselves through the appreciative eyes of others. Most people are their own worst critics, never truly recognizing their inner and outer beauty. This charm is designed to increase your awareness of positive personal attributes, and to accentuate those to the people you meet or care about.

You will need a small mirror (the size of a compact) and four tiny tumbled cat's eye stones that have a flat side. During a waxing moon, go out into the night and glue the four stones on the mirror at the four compass points. As you place each one, repeat the appropriate incantation:

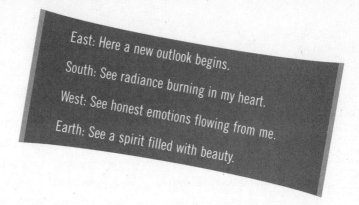

East: Here a new outlook begins.

South: See radiance burning in my heart.

West: See honest emotions flowing from me.

Earth: See a spirit filled with beauty.

Keep this nearby as often as possible. When you feel your self-esteem slipping, or others' opinions of you are hurtful, look into the mirror and see the truth.

Alternative Components:

Take love foods with you each day for lunch to internalize and welcome love. Possibilities include peaches, plums, raspberries, and tomatoes. Wear more pink or red clothing and carry stones like pink tourmaline or rhodocrosite so that you vibrate with loving energy.

To draw love into your life, work during a waxing to full moon, on Fridays, during the month of June, or when the moon is in Scorpio.

Prosperous Pockets

Money may not buy happiness, but it certainly makes being unhappy a lot easier to live with! These bits of portable magic are, therefore, designed to increase the abundance in your life. It should be noted, however, that prosperity is not always measured in dollars and cents. It is also found in plentiful joy, health, and peace.

To help draw prosperity and wealth your way, call on Tyche, the Greek goddess whose very name means "fortune." Alternatively, consider Erzulie, a generous Haitian goddess who bestows wealth on those in need.

THE SEEDS OF SUCCESS:

Seeds appear in many old spells for prosperity, because they symbolize growth and the land's providence (which used to be directly linked to wealth). Building on this foundation, get some dried alfalfa sprouts, pumpkin seeds, and popcorn, as well as a portable container for them. Empower the seeds under a full moon (for full pockets), saying,

What I sow will root and grow:
these seeds are my prosperity;

these seeds are my abundance;
these seeds are Tyche's providence.

When you need extra cash quickly, take one of each seed and toss them out to the earth as if sowing grain. Then watch for opportunity to knock.

FOOL'S GOLD:

In Mexico, pyrite is considered a powerful token for drawing money. Put two pieces of pyrite on your altar or entertainment center with a green candle. Carve a dollar sign on the candle, then light it, saying,

Erzulie, answer my need,
constraints be freed,
today I claim prosperity.

Let the candle burn out naturally. Leave one stone in your home to keep providence there, and carry the other with you to attract improved finances.

OUR DAILY BREAD:

As the staff of life, bread is considered a potent symbol of prosperity. Never cut your bread, or you will cut off your abundance. Gently tear it instead.

Gypsies tell us that carrying a small piece of bread in our pockets acts as an amulet against poverty. To reinforce this even further, put your hands over the bread to bless it, saying,

*From the earth's bounty, I receive
and welcome the energy of abundance.*

Eat half of the bread. Wrap the rest in a scrap of white cloth or a napkin, and put it in your pocket. If the bread ever crumbles, give it to the land as an offering, then make a new amulet. The breaking disperses the energy, and the birds will carry your wishes on their wings.

THE BUZZ:

Victorian people regarded bees as messengers between heaven and earth, and they often wore bee jewelry as charms to bring improved finances (probably associated with the honey market). Or they donned fish pendants for profuseness. Either of these adornments can still work today in the form of pins, tie tacks, rings, and so on.

Take the chosen charm and leave it in the sunlight for as long as you wish to encourage divine blessing. Then, each time you put it on, say,

> *Within the binding of this pin*
> *so Tyche's magic shall begin.*
> *Let fortune find and bring to me*
> *a pocket of prosperity.*

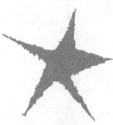

Wear this on days when you need a little extra money (or the opportunity to make some) to come your way.

PARSLEY PROTECTION:

Put a piece of parsley or dried lettuce in your wallet. As you do, recite this incantation nine times:

> *Less goes out than goes in;*
> *Erzulie's magic here begins.*
> *Prosperity within remains and grows,*
> *to ease my cash flow woes.*

If possible, repeat the incantation each time you open your wallet (mentally or verbally) so that no excess goes out, and more money returns.

MAGNETIC APPEAL:

Take a magnet and attach it to a dollar bill using green thread. As you wrap the thread around the bill and the magnet, repeat this incantation until the thread is totally secured:

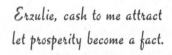

Erzulie, cash to me attract
let prosperity become a fact.

Carry this with you regularly to draw money to you.

THE MONEY TREE:

When I was a child, my mother used to make these for my birthday. They consisted of a small branch, secured in clay, to which coins and bills were attached by ribbon and tape. You can make your own magical money tree. Simply adhere quarters and bills to a branch whenever you have a little extra to spare. As you put the money on the tree, say,

Wherever this goes, money grows!

When you need a little extra cash fast, take one of the coins or bills off the tree and either use it or carry it with you to attract more money.

Alternative Components:

Use anything gold, silver, or green (all of which are associated with money). Wear or burn prosperous aromatics like almond or banana. Carry money-attracting stones like aventurine, bloodstone, and jet. Bless your bank cards, checkbooks, and calculators.

Work in the sunlight or on Sundays to encourage more gold in your life. A waxing to full moon helps money grow, as does the month of May and a moon in Virgo. The moon in Libra emphasizes making a profit, while Thursdays are fortunate for all financial transactions.

Having It All

We all wish for lives filled with contentment, health, happiness, and prosperity. There is nothing wrong with wanting the best for ourselves and those we love. The idea behind pocket magic is to create the vibration of success and then take that energy with you everywhere you go. This fetish, therefore, is designed to be a general all-purpose power center that you can energize and draw from as needed.

THE WISHING WELL:

Take any large bowl. Drip a few drops of different-colored candle wax in the bottom of the bowl, then adhere a white candle to that spot. The different colors represent diverse needs and goals, while the white binds this variety together in harmony. Each morning, light the candle when you get up and put a coin in the bowl. Make your wish for the day. Blow out the candle before you leave the house.

Whenever you desperately need to have a wish fulfilled, remove a coin from the bowl and either plant it in rich soil or throw it into moving water so that your message of need will be carried through the earth. When the bowl is filled with coins, use all but a few (these "seeds" always remain in your bowl) for random acts of kindness, like getting treats for the neighborhood kids or helping a homeless person. Your generosity will return to you threefold to keep the magic of benevolence, both mundane and divine, with you always.

THE LAST WORD

My husband will be the first to tell you that I always have a few last comments on any matter. My parting thoughts for this book can be summed up in three words: magic is everywhere. It's in the sunrise, the laughter of children, inspired art, and even insects (the flying kind, not your last blind date). Most important, magic is in *you*. Even when absolutely no components are handy, don't forget that you already have what you need to withdraw the Goddess's power from your heart's pocket—faith and love. So, go for it!

ACKNOWLEDGMENTS

My thanks for this book begins at home with my husband, Paul, for believing in my unique spiritual vision. Additional appreciation goes to Jenny for helping me find a terrific publisher, Caroline for rallying behind the idea for this book, and Sally for acting as a trustworthy courier. You four are the stepparents for these pages.